M000288628

Rahul K. Nath, MD

Founder and Medical Director
Texas Nerve and Paralysis Institute
Houston, Texas

OBSTETRIC BRACHIAL PLEXUS INJURIES

ERB'S PALSY

The Nath Method of Diagnosis and Treatment

Illustrated by
Marjon Fatemizadeh-Aucoin

This book is intended as an informational resource only for caregivers, families and patients suffering from brachial plexus nerve injuries. No attempt to provide specific medical advice is intended. It is not intended to infer that surgery is always the best choice for a given brachial plexus nerve injury. You should always contact a specialist directly for diagnosis and treatment of your specific problem, and a second opinion is always a good idea.

"Obstetric Brachial Plexus Injuries," by Rahul K. Nath, MD. ISBN 978-1-58939-970-9.

Library of Congress data on file with publisher.

Published 2007 by Virtualbookworm.com Publishing Inc., P.O. Box 9949, College Station, TX 77842, US. ©2006/2007, Dr. Rahul K. Nath. All rights reserved. No part of this publication may be reproduced, stored in a retrieval system, or transmitted in any form or by any means, electronic, mechanical, recording or otherwise, without the prior written permission of Dr. Rahul K. Nath.

Manufactured in the United States of America.

This book is dedicated…

to my parents, Surrendra and Sushila (I hope you feel better soon, Dad.)
to my wife Usha (nothing happens without you)
to my children, Priya and Devin (the best ever)
to Joginder and Bala (also the best)
to Dr. Krishna Kumar and Shubha Kumar (both inspirations).

…I love you all

This book was written in collaboration with:

Dr. Kim L. Farina
Dr. Melia Paizi
Sonya E. Melcher

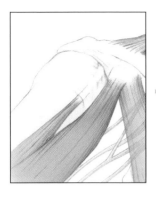

Preface

The Nath Method of Treatment of brachial plexus injuries in the newborn has arisen out of my experience of over 10 years and 5,000 patients. It relies on understanding the anatomic and physiologic bases for the most common abnormalities of function that arise from these injuries. Since the deformities that do arise are predictable given the nerves that are involved, it is most logical to present the basic scientific facts as a prelude to critically discussing management. I believe that knowing the root cause of a particular problem will allow a more comprehensive understanding of the reasons for a given treatment plan, rather than accepting it blindly. Clinical management consists of diagnosis and treatment and these will be discussed together, in Chapter 5, within the context of a simple question-and-answer format that should allow a clearer vision of how all the involved elements are integrated.

I have purposely kept the format simple and brief. The long-term plan is to add components to the initial monograph so that it will constantly evolve to reflect the most modern information and treatment protocols.

The overall perspective presented is a very personal one and does reflect my views on a very diverse field; others may disagree with some or all of what is presented. I believe that everything I do or say is based on the strongest evidence available. Everything is based on my own experience with management of several thousand patients as well as my observations of those managed by other doctors and centers.

I hope that this book will be useful to a wide variety of interested parties, and that the overall impact will be to improve the quality of life of children and adults who have suffered this injury. Many protocols presented are simple and straightforward and will allow application of the management plans to patients in developing countries where treatment is often not attempted because of the daunting complexity of some traditional surgical and therapeutic measures.

The overall theme of this book is simplicity. Far too many words on brachial plexus injury have been written and spoken based on inadequate information. It has been my experience that simple solutions offer the best results. I believe that the available evidence bears out this truth.

One keystone of my treatment protocols is the understanding that the shoulder is the most commonly affected element of the extremity and that effective management of the shoulder is critical to the overall outcome of limb function. The placement of the hand in space and the direction of biceps and triceps action are all influenced directly by the development and health of the shoulder.

Several additional important points regarding shoulder function are: (1) **Vertical** restrictions of movement are related to the presence of **soft tissue** abnormalities. Contractures in the latissimus dorsi, teres major, pectoralis and other muscles of the axilla and chest are formed and adduction deformity of the shoulder is the result. Surgical management is required in significant cases and is aimed at release and transfer of contracted muscles. (2) **Horizontal** restrictions of shoulder movement are related to the presence of **bony** abnormalities. Elevation and abnormal lateral rotation of the scapula develops due to rhomboid weakness and medial rotation of the humerus and arm is the result. Surgical management is required in significant cases and is aimed at release of the humerus from the abnormally placed scapula. (3) The Scapula forms the cornerstone of glenohumeral joint development and health. An abnormally-situated scapula will influence the position and function of the arm and hand and result in severe developmental abnormalities of the joint. Treatment must be aimed at the scapula and its relationship to the humeral head within the glenoid fossa.

The impact of a major nerve injury on the developing limb cannot be underestimated, and the long-term sequelae of early derangements of growth are predictable and severe. The natural corollary of this statement is that early therapeutic and surgical intervention should result in improved adult quality of function and life. That is perhaps the most important message of this book, and I believe that long-term tracking of such patients will prove this statement.

I will welcome suggestions and comments for improving the contents and layout of the book. The current version does not contain detailed therapy and electrical stimulation information, but my experience has certainly been that both are critically important to achieve the best outcomes in patients with nerve injury. Future editions of the book will devote significantly more space to detailed descriptions of these modalities.

I would also like to point out the valuable resources available at my website: **www.drnathbrachialplexus.com,** including links to volunteers who have been through the processes and obstacles of dealing with a brachial plexus injury in their child:

> **http://www.drnathbrachialplexus.com/vnu/index.php**
> **http://www.drnathbrachialplexus.com/forum**

Rahul K. Nath, MD
Houston, Texas, USA

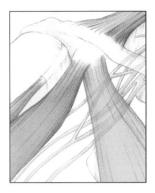

Foreword

Brachial plexus injuries in the newborn are as diverse as the individual infants themselves. This is obvious when the anatomy of the brachial plexus is examined and seen to be as complex as any anatomical area in the human body. However, certain patterns do arise and if identified, can allow simplified diagnosis and, ultimately, treatment. The key to management of these injuries is pattern recognition. After that, therapeutic and surgical plans can be picked from a menu of available choices that suit the particular child and his or her patterns.

The structure of this book is therefore designed to present the anatomy the common patterns and the treatments that will benefit the large majority of affected children. An interested caregiver will come to understand and appreciate how anatomy dictates function and how restoration of anatomy is the key to good outcomes. Since anatomy is the basis for management, it will be apparent that certain such derangements are amenable to therapy and others are not. Unlike weakness, stiffness and abnormal motor patterns, contractures and bony deformities are not amenable to therapy alone.

All the elements of weakness, stiffness, abnormal movements, contractures and bony deformities can be expected and predicted in this population of patients because of one important fact: children at the time of birth grow at an exponential rate. Since growth is influenced by nerve supply, it is logical that growth impairment occurs with nerve injury in children, especially younger ones. In an adult, without growth issues, this degree of nerve injury might be trivial in many cases. In a newborn, even relatively minor nerve injuries will exact a toll in extremity growth and development. Another important factor is the asymmetry of nerve injury: usually the upper part of the brachial plexus is injured, while the lower part is less affected, resulting in asymmetric development of the extremity. This is what leads to contractures and bony deformities and an understanding of this point allows effective management of the injury.

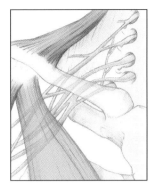

Table of Contents

Chapter 1 Nerve Injuries & Their Management

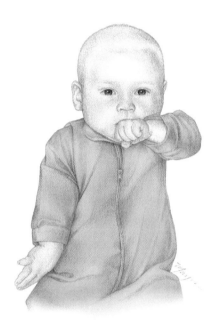

Introduction

The brachial plexus is the most complex peripheral neural unit. It supplies the arm and hand, allowing expression of the mind through writing, art, athletic endeavor and delicate manipulation of the environment. Injuries to the plexus, therefore, have consequences far beyond the structural damage involved. The significance of injury can best be appreciated by understanding the layers of complexity within the brachial plexus at anatomic as well as functional levels.

This chapter serves as an introduction to the physiologic role of the brachial plexus within the functioning of the entire body. It will also hopefully be an entry point into understanding the consequences of derangements of the nerves comprising the brachial plexus in the context of growth and development of the child sustaining injury to the plexus.

It will become apparent that although the birth injury in the newborn occurs to the nerves, the main adverse events that follow from that initial injury involve the muscles, bones and joints of the affected extremity. The natural place to begin a study of injury to the brachial plexus is at the structural anatomy, an overview of which follows.

General Discussion

Nerves

Neuroanatomy

The human nervous system is subdivided into the central and peripheral systems. The central system is composed of the brain and the spinal column, from which thirty one pairs of spinal nerves emerge. For classification purposes, the spine is divided into cervical, thoracic, lumbar and sacral regions. Spinal nerve pairs are grouped as follows: eight cervical, twelve thoracic, five lumbar, five sacral and one coccygeal. Each spinal nerve is associated with an efferent ventral (anterior) and an afferent dorsal (posterior) root (Figure 1.1). Efferent (motor) neurons carry impulses originating in the central nervous system towards the periphery. Afferent (sensory) neurons carry impulses originating on peripheral sensory receptors towards the central nervous system. The cell bodies of ventral root nerves are located within the gray matter of the central nervous system. Dorsal roots are associated with a ganglion, an ovoid enlargement in which neuronal cell bodies reside. Ganglion cell bodies

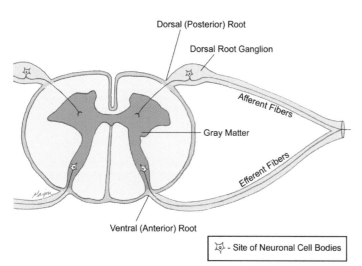

Figure 1.1. Transverse section of the spinal column. Efferent motor neurons stem from the ventral root of the spinal nerve with cell bodies located within the gray matter of the cord. The cell bodies of the afferent fibers are located within a ganglion that is distal from the dorsal root of the spinal nerve.

are bipolar and give off a medial and lateral fiber. Medial fibers extend into the spine to form the actual dorsal root of the spinal nerve. Lateral fibers, on the other hand, make their way to peripheral somatic receptors.

The Motor Neuron

A basic understanding of microscopic peripheral nerve anatomy is necessary to understand obstetric brachial plexus injuries (OBPI) and the development of their treatment plans. Individual motor neurons originate with the cell body in the anterior horn of the spinal cord and travel through the body with an elongated axon to the muscles they innervate. The nucleus of the neuron is located within the cell body. Individual neurons are bundled together, in a highly organized manner, with connective and nutritive tissues to form nerves that traverse the body[1, 2].

Each neuronal axon is bounded by its own membrane, the axolemma. The axolemma contains ion channels that maintain the cell's membrane potential and propagate the action potential. Several Schwann cells will contact an axon along its length. In the case of myelinated axons, Schwann cells provide an insulating sheath of myelin by wrapping around the axon in a spiral fashion. Myelinated axons are capable of rapid action potential conduction. Unmyelinated axons are also in contact with Schwann cells, though more tangentially and without the layers of myelin insulation. The long motor neurons are typically myelinated, while short and interneuronal axons are often unmyelinated. Each of these myelinated nerve fibers, or group of unmyelinated nerve fibers is then surrounded by the endoneurium, made chiefly of collagen fibers[1, 2].

Nerve fibers travel along the nerve bundled into groups called fascicles. The bundled nerves are seated in additional connective tissue, called the perineurium. The perineurial tissue provides the nerve with the majority of its tensile strength[3]. The trunks of the brachial plexus are composed of roughly 55% perineurial connective tissue[4]. A nerve may contain a single fascicle (monofascicular), a few (2-10) fascicles (oligofascicular), or many (more than 10) fascicles (polyfascicular)[1, 2]. This organization can change over the length of a nerve. Surrounding the organized fascicles is the epineurium. Where nerves pass over or through joints, connective tissues of the epineurium take up an increased proportion of the nerve's cross-section, protecting the fascicles from excessive pressure or friction. The epineurium is continuous with a sheath of loosely organized tissue, the mesoneurium, which contacts surrounding soft tissue, including blood vessels, and allows nerves to glide during movement.

Nerve Injury and Healing

In functioning motor nerves, an electrical signal is conducted down the length of the axon to reach the motor end plate where it triggers the release of acetylcholine. Injury to the nerve fiber can affect nerve function by interrupting or impeding axonal conduction. This effectively reduces or prevents communication to distal musculature. Injury that disrupts communication between the cell body and distal portions of its axon stimulates Wallerian degeneration distal to the site of the injury. The extent of injury has been usefully classified and described by Seddon, Sunderland, and Mackinnon [2, 5, 6] (Table 1.I, Figure 1.2).

The mildest class of injury, called neurapraxia by Seddon and first degree (I) by Sunderland, is a conduction block where the nerve is in-continuity and Wallerian degeneration of distal portions of the axon does not take place. Recovery from this first degree injury is expected within three months.

In second degree injuries (Sunderland II), axons are no longer continuous, though the nerve itself remains intact, and will attempt to regenerate through axon sprouting. Distal to the second degree injury, Wallerian degeneration

takes place. Healing requires nerve regeneration between the site of injury and the distal end of the nerve. Time of recovery depends on the distance to be covered, averaging 1 inch per month. Therefore, proximal injuries (those closer to the spinal cord) will have farther to travel during regeneration and will require more time to heal than a more distal injury. A related concept is that infants and children will tend to have a faster recovery than adults due in part to the shorter distances that need to be traversed for effective regeneration through to the motor end plates.

A third degree injury (Sunderland III) similar to the second degree injury, but during healing, excessive scarring of the endoneurium, the fine innermost connective tissue covering individual nerve fibers, occurs, and this hinders axon regeneration. Recovery will take place at less than 1 inch per month where it is slowed by the scar tissue. The degree of recovery is determined by the degree of scarring as well as which particular fascicles are affected.

In more severe injuries, recovery is not expected without surgical intervention. The nerve is still in-continuity in a fourth degree injury as defined by Sunderland. There is, however, scar build up to such an extent that a significant percentage of nerve regeneration is blocked. Surgical intervention is required to reestablish nerve transduction by removing the scar tissue and reconnecting proximal and distal nerve segments directly or with a nerve graft. Second, third and fourth degree injuries as defined by Sunderland

Table 1.I *Classifications of Nerve Injury*

	Sunderland	Seddon	Description of Injury	Recovery Period
Mildest	I	Neurapraxia	Conduction block, nerve is in-continuity, Wallerian degeneration does not take place	≤ 3 months
	II	Axonotmesis	Axon not continuous, nerve itself remains intact, axonal sprouting, Wallerian degeneration	1 inch per month
	III		During healing, excessive scarring of the endoneurium occurs that hinders axon regeneration	< 1 inch per month where it is slowed by the scar tissue; determined by degree of scarring and involved fascicles
	IV		Nerve is still in-continuity, scar build up blocks nerve regeneration	Surgical intervention required to re-establish nerve transduction by removing scar tissue and reconnecting nerve segments
Most Severe	V	Neurotmesis	Rupture of the nerve, it is no longer a continuous fiber	Recovery requires surgical intervention

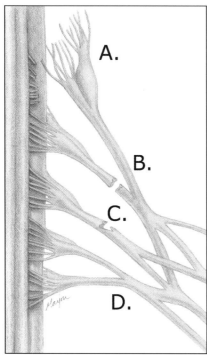

Figure 1.2. Common types of nerve injury.
A. Avulsion. B. Rupture. C. Partial Rupture D. Stretch Injury, nerve remains in-continuity.

ent portions of the brachial plexus are injured to differing degrees. Each individual nerve can also be injured in a complex fashion. Accurate electrodiagnosis of this type of injury is difficult, and a careful clinical examination is necessary for a more accurate diagnosis and prognosis.

In my experience, the majority of brachial plexus injuries in the newborn are stretch injuries without rupture or avulsion, degree I-II in the Sunderland scale. This is recent knowledge implied from treatment outcomes of the muscle and bony deformities that flow from the initial nerve injury.

Brachial Plexus: Anatomy of the Injury

Brachial Plexus Anatomy

The brachial plexus is a complex network of nerves beginning with 5 roots in the spinal cord (anterior branches of the spinal nerves) combining into 3 trunks (upper, middle and lower) and then bifurcating and regrouping into 3 cords (lateral with contributions from the upper and middle trunks, posterior with contributions from all three trunks, and medial with nerves from only the lower trunk) (Figures 1.3-1.4). Along the way, nerves branch from the roots, trunk, and cords. The collection of nerves originating in the brachial plexus innervates the shoulder, arm, elbow, wrist, hand, and fingers[1, 7, 8].

The five brachial plexus nerve roots are named C5, C6, C7, C8, and T1 after the cervical vertebrae from which they emerge. The C5-C7 roots emerge from above the vertebrae with the same name while C8 and T1 emerge from above and below the T1 vertebra, respectively. C5 and C6 roots combine to form the upper trunk, the most frequent site of birth injury. C7 comprises the middle trunk, and C8 and T1 are the lower roots which combine to form the lower trunk (Figure 1.5).

Birth Injury

The rate of obstetric brachial plexus injury in the United States appears to be fairly constant at a rate of 0.38-2.6 per 1000 births[9-12]. The most common risk factor in the occurrence of an obstetric brachial plexus injury is shoulder dystocia, a situation where there is, presumably, a mismatch between the maternal pelvic diameter and the size of the infant's body and shoulders[1,13]. Shoulder dystocia is more

were grouped together as axonotmesis by Seddon since the injuries show functional loss and yet nerve continuity is maintained.

In contrast, a fifth degree[6] injury, or neurotmesis[5], describes a rupture or avulsion of the nerve. Due to excessive stretching forces or to mechanical transection, the nerve is no longer a continuous unit. Ruptured nerves, torn distal to the spinal column, have a chance of healing if the gap between proximal and distal segments is short. Recovery usually requires surgical intervention to repair the gap left between proximal and distal nerve segments. Avulsion is a form of neurotmesis transection in which the nerve root is torn from the spinal cord. Nerves torn from the spinal cord have no chance of regeneration, as the tissue of the spinal cord does not regenerate. A related concept is that nerve reconstruction by direct repair or graft in avulsion injury is generally not considered effective.

Mackinnon has described a sixth degree injury, also called neuroma in-continuity, that manifests as differing degrees of injury to individual fascicles[2, 3]. Since the injury is mixed, so is the recovery. This is a useful concept when considering treatment options for obstetric brachial plexus injuries. In obstetric brachial plexus injuries, all degrees of injury are possible, and often there is a mixed pattern in which differ-

common with above average birth-weight babies, but this is not always the case.

The uppermost roots (C5-C6) tend to bear the brunt of the injury and because of their more superficial location in the neck, are more vulnerable to injury. In severe cases, lower root injury may accompany stretching of C5 and C6. Lower roots may be injured to a greater extent because of the angle at which the roots leave the spinal column and travel down the neck[15-17]. Associated injuries may include fracture of the clavicle or humerus, and humeral dislocation.

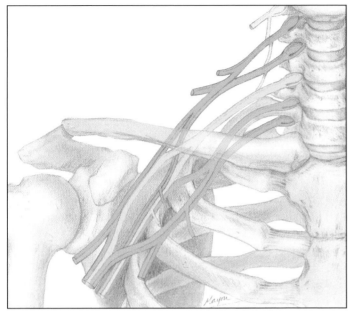

Figure 1.3. The Brachial Plexus. The brachial plexus stems from five spinal nerves and innervates the musculature of the shoulder, arm and hand.

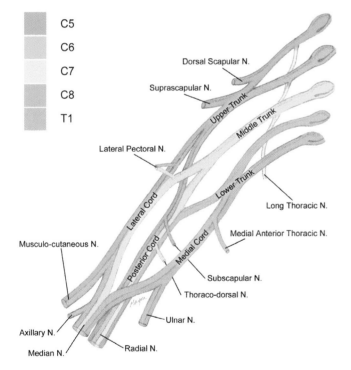

C5
C6
C7
C8
T1

Dorsal Scapular N.
Suprascapular N.
Upper Trunk
Middle Trunk
Lateral Pectoral N.
Lower Trunk
Lateral Cord
Long Thoracic N.
Musculo-cutaneous N.
Posterior Cord
Medial Cord
Medial Anterior Thoracic N.
Subscapular N.
Thoraco-dorsal N.
Ulnar N.
Axillary N.
Radial N.
Median N.

Figure 1.4. Anatomy of the Brachial Plexus. The roots from which the brachial plexus originates emerge from the spinal cord, merge and divide into the upper (C5-C6), middle (C7) and lower (C8-T1) trunks of the brachial plexus. Each of the three trunks further divides into anterior and posterior divisions. The anterior division of the upper and middle trunks form the lateral cord, the anterior division of the lower trunk forms the medial cord and all of the posterior divisions unite to form the medial cord. From these cords stem the nerve pathways that control shoulder and upper extremity function.

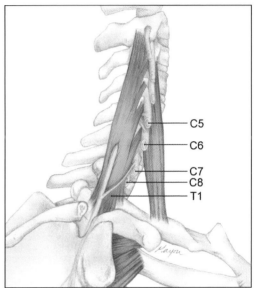

Figure 1.5. The nerve roots of the brachial plexus are named after the vertebrae from which they emerge. Note that the vulnerable uppermost root (C5-C6) is the most superficial and is under the most tension, while the deeper position of the lower roots and the decreased tension that they are under, protects them from injury.

Brachial plexus injuries that occur during breech deliveries may have a different mechanism of onset, and are more likely to be bilateral. Although avulsions of the upper roots are more likely during breech than during vertex delivery, the most common injury is to the C5 and C6 roots without involvement of the other roots[15, 17, 18]. Brachial plexus injuries may also occur, although very rarely, during cesarean sections.

Unlike adults, children may have complications from even the most simple nerve injury due to the growth issues that are present (Figure 1.6). The mildest and most common OBPI is neurapraxia; the most severe is avulsion[1, 19]. Both types of injury have the potential to result in permanent disability.

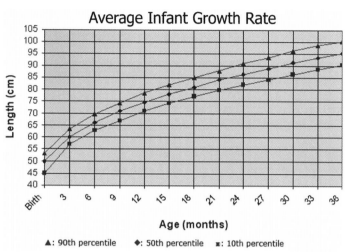

Average Infant Growth Rate

▲: 90th percentile   ◆: 50th percentile   ■: 10th percentile

Figure 1.6. Rapid growth that occurs during early development contributes to secondary and tertiary effects of OBPI.

The Nath Method

Management

Surgery to reconstruct the injured nerves is not recommended for neurapraxic injuries, but early surgical intervention is considered when avulsion is definitively diagnosed. In between these extremes is a continuum of injuries that will

heal in a variety of circumstances. In most cases, children will benefit from management that conservatively treats the nerve injury and focuses on the upper muscle and bone consequences that often occur.

Although each individual infant and brachial plexus injury is unique, abnormal movement patterns may be defined by following large numbers of injured children throughout their development. A thorough understanding of these patterns is important in making decisions about how and when to treat children with OBPI. The primary goal is always to improve the child's quality of life by restoring function, while balancing aggressive management with a respect for the body's ability to repair the injury spontaneously. The task is made easier by understanding that common deformities such as muscle contractures and bony derangements do not spontaneously resolve, while nerve injuries generally do.

Nerve Healing/Recovery of OBPI

The neural systems of infants are still developing and their nerve networks possess a natural ability to recover and adapt. The connective tissue within the nerve structure also allows for some axial loading without disruption of the contained axons. In addition, the complex networking of nerves within the brachial plexus may contribute to recovery because of its inherent redundancy.

There are many techniques that take advantage of this adaptability to maximize recovery without the need for surgical intervention. The decision of whether to surgically repair the nerves, however, does typically need to be made in the first 6 months of life. Nerves heal at a rate of 1 inch

Table 1.II *Narakas Classification of Brachial Plexus Injury Based on Clinical Observations*

Group	Newborn Clinical Presentation	Typical Recovery	Probable Lesion (Sunderland Degree)
1	absence of abduction, external rotation, elbow flexion, forearm supination	recovery begins within 1 month; full recovery by 4-6 months	I and II to the upper trunk
2	similar to group 1 with weaker active elbow extension	≥ 1 month before recovery of shoulder and elbow flexion, steady improvement but likely development of contractures that limit motion	II and III to the upper trunk, I and II to C7 root
3	flail shoulder, absence of elbow flexion, weak extension, flexed wrist, closed fist	slow partial recovery of up to 15 months; weak, limited function and secondary deformities likely	IV and V to upper trunk, III and IV to C7 root
4	flail extremity, half-open hand, little finger movement	poor shoulder function; arm rests in abduction, elbow flexion, internal rotation, supinated forearm; absence of external rotation	variety of severe lesions (II through IV) involving upper, middle and lower trunks

per month and supplied muscles will terminally atrophy if not reinnervated by about 12 to 18 months of life. The longer a required nerve repair is delayed, the lower the ceiling of final outcome will be. Delay beyond a year to 18 months generally results in permanent paralysis that will require more complex reconstruction with nerve transfers and free functional muscle transfers.

Recovery from injury depends on the degree of nerve injury and the pattern of nerve injury. If the injury is contained to the upper plexus and is neurapraxic in nature, secondary reconstruction of deformities generally has good potential for restoration of position and movement. Injury to the lower roots that results in loss of continuity of nerve structure will have significantly greater morbidity, will require more heroic reconstructive methods, and will result in greater shortening and physical deformity of the extremity. Most commonly, the upper roots are affected due to their more superficial position in the neck while the lower roots are protected by their deeper position and inherent laxity as they exit the spinal column.

Classification of Injury

Location/Patterns of Injury

Clinical examination determines which muscles are paralyzed, and thus, which brachial plexus nerve roots are affected. Narakas defined four main classifications of increasingly severe injury based on clinical observations[19] (Table 1.II). Classification of brachial plexus injuries by nerve root injury is a useful tool for predicting future recovery patterns and identifying potential treatment options. Typical birth injuries involve the upper roots alone, the upper and middle together or upper, middle and lower. It is extremely rare (<1%) for an obstetric brachial plexus injury to involve only the lower roots [20] (Klumpke's paralysis), and was, therefore, not included in Narakas's classification system.

Injuries to the upper trunk fall into Narakas Group 1, and are equivalent to Erb's palsy in which C5 and C6 roots undergo a mild stretch, consistent with a Sunderland degree injury of I-II[19]. Partial recovery is expected within the first three months, and excellent nerve function is eventually seen in the majority of this group. However, it is critical to note that a recovered nerve injury in the infant population still may produce significant morbidity due to muscle imbalances and bony deformities that result from the typically asymmetric injury occurring at a time of rapid

limb growth. Even seemingly trivial injuries cannot be predicted to result in complete recovery of function, and muscle and bony derangements may occur in up to half of all injured babies.

In more severe C5-C6 injuries, the nerves are ruptured or avulsed[21]. Clinical evaluation of the newborn's arm posture will typically show medial rotation at the shoulder (due to paralysis of the infraspinatus, teres minor and supraspinatus), a pronated forearm (due to paralysis of the supinator muscle and biceps brachii), and an extended elbow (due to paralysis of the biceps brachii and brachialis in the face of a strong triceps muscle). Additionally, paralysis of the deltoid and supraspinatus results in loss of shoulder abduction[8, 19]. An injury of the proximal C5-C6 roots will also result in weakness of the rhomboid and serratus anterior muscles. The clinical manifestations will develop as scapular winging and elevation and rotation of the scapula (the SHEAR deformity, see Chs. 3-4).

Note that the manifestations of a Narakas Group 1 injury may develop a similar clinical presentation to complete avulsion of the upper roots due to the secondary effects of the initial nerve injury on growth. This occurs because "co-contraction" may exist in opposing muscle groups due to the asymmetry of the typical brachial plexus injury. Commonly, co-contractions happen in two situations: (1) Shoulder abductors and external rotators versus the shoulder internal rotators and adductors. Here, the loss of abduction and external rotation is due to delayed recovery of these muscles (supplied by the injured C5 root), compared to the intact internal rotators/adductors, that mimics complete paralysis due to rupture/avulsion of the C5 root. (2) Elbow flexors versus extensors. Here, the loss of biceps flexion is due to delayed recovery of the biceps and medial brachialis (supplied by the injured C5-C6 nerve roots) compared to the intact triceps (supplied by the intact C7). Lack of elbow flexion in this circumstance mimics complete C6 injury by rupture or avulsion.

Both co-contraction situations are distinguishable from a true complete injury to the upper roots by preoperative and/or intra-operative electromyography (EMG) testing. In the case of a co-contraction, EMG will show the presence of functional motor units in the biceps and affected shoulder muscles, indicating recovery that is masked by overly strong opposing muscle groups that were relatively spared in the initial injury. The ideal situation for precise EMG testing is in the context of an operating or minor procedure room where sedation is offered by a licensed anesthesiologist. The presence of fibrillation potentials in the paraspinal muscles is a sign of severe injury and these tend to require reconstruction of the nerves involved. In my experience, nerve transfers are preferable to nerve grafting although both have a good record of success in this population when performed appropriately.

Narakas Group 2 injury involves the C7 root with the degree of injury to C5-C6 typically increased to Sunderland degree II-III. This type of injury results in weaker elbow extension than seen in Group 1 due to the C7 injury[18]. Since both upper and middle trunk roots are involved, these children virtually always develop significant secondary and tertiary effects, which clinically present as persistent medial rotation of the arm and adduction at the shoulder. These positions are related to contracture formation on axillary and chest muscles (causing adduction) and abnormal positioning of the scapula and other bony elements of the SHEAR deformity (causing medial rotation) (for more on this, see Chs. 2-3).

By following the recovery pattern, Narakas Groups 1 and 2 can be distinguished at about 6 weeks. The arm presentation of group 2 will be similar to that observed in Group 1, but with a slight flex to the elbow due to weakened extension. Additionally, the wrist and fingers may be flexed. This is called the "waiter's tip" position of the arm and hand (Figure 1.7). Taken together, Group 1 and 2 upper root palsies are the most common, accounting for approximately 75% of reported cases[22].

When all the trunks are injured, the effects are seen in the entire arm and hand. In the Narakas Group 3 injury, C5-C6 injury is consistent with Degrees IV-V Sunderland injury[19]. C7 is probably injured to Degree III and C8-T1 injuries to Degrees I-II. Because the forces required to injure all five roots are very significant, there is also a greater likelihood that at least some of the roots will be avulsed in these injuries.

Infants with Narakas Group 3 injury present with a flail arm and hand, and there will be no sensibility in the arm. In most cases, the hand will recover function slowly, if at all. Because the distance from the site of plexus injury in the neck to the target organ of the hand is significant, the final outcome will be delayed and will not be as good as an equivalent injury to the upper roots. Additionally, the delicate intrinsic muscles of the hand are extremely sensitive to denervation and, therefore, an injury to their supplying T1 root will limit final outcome. The shoulder and biceps will tend to recover very slowly, the deltoid may take up to a year to regain function and internal rotation will persist. As muscles are reinnervated in an asymmetric fashion, muscle imbalances occur in the shoulder that will virtually always lead to bone deformations in this group.

It is worth mentioning that there are subgroups of patients within this particular population that present with unusual patterns of deformity:

(1) Some patients recover shoulder abduction almost completely but maintain a persistent medial rotation posture due to the presence of a SHEAR deformity. In these patients, there are minimal to no contractures present in the axilla and chest, yet there is lateralization and elevation of the scapula, probably due to persistent injury of the dorsal scapular nerve, rendering the rhomboid weak. Treatment of the SHEAR deformity is performed as outlined in Chapters 3-4.

(2) Some patients have relative sparing of the dorsal scapular nerve but co-contraction of the shoulder muscles occurs. These patients exhibit lack of shoulder abduction but maintain a neutral position of the arm. Treatment of the axillary and chest contractures is performed as outlined in Chapter 2.

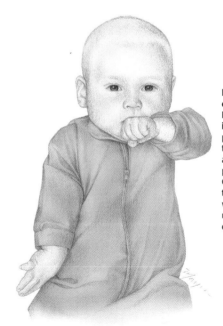

Figure 1.7. Clinical presentation of infants with Narakas Group 1 and 2 injuries. Patients typically present with medial rotation, forearm pronation and elbow extension. The patient pictured here has a Group 2 injury, evident by the waiter's tip position in which the palm faces upward and the hand projects distally.

(3) A third group of patients presents with medial rotation posturing of the humerus combined with a supination deformity of the forearm. The two deformities "cancel out" at the hand giving the false impression of neutral positioning of the limb (see text box on Arm Rotated Medially with Supination deformity, Ch. 3). In actuality, the elbow crease is not visible, indicating loss of neutral position of the upper arm, while the neutral-appearing position of the hand indicates the second deformity, an excessive, fixed supination posture of the forearm. Treatment is aimed at correcting the SHEAR deformity that causes the medial rotation of the humerus, and at the fixed forearm supination. Both must be addressed by bony surgery. The specific nerve injury leading to this pattern is not known, but may be one that relatively spares C6 while injuring C5, C7 and C8.

The most severe group of injuries is Narakas Group 4. All three trunks are affected with probable avulsions of C8 and/or C7 and rupture of C5 and sometimes C6. A wide variety of lesions are seen during surgical exploration of these injuries[19]. The most extreme cases, in which multiple roots are ruptured or avulsed, are best helped by nerve graft or transfer. There is also the possible presence of a Horner's sign (ptosis, lighter iris and pupil that fails to dilate in dark) that indicates the injury to the lower roots is close to the spinal cord and is most likely to be an avulsion. There will probably be no spontaneous recovery from these injuries.

Degree/Severity/Type of OBPI Injury

The severity of injury to the brachial plexus can range from neurapraxia (stretch) to neurotmesis (rupture). The ruptures may be more severe if they occur near the spinal cord. Several nerves branch from the roots and proximal trunks of the brachial plexus, and examination of the muscles they innervate can help identify probable avulsions.

Neurapraxic injury results when the stretching forces are not great enough to rupture the affected nerve(s). Nerves that retain continuity heal more quickly and completely than nerves that are fully or partially ruptured.

Neurapraxia will generally resolve itself in a matter of months since the nerve fiber remains intact. Nevertheless, secondary and tertiary effects to muscle and bone development should be expected in a significant percentage of such patients.

Ruptured axons will grow back at a rate of 1mm/day until the new growth crosses the gap in the nerve created by the nerve injury. Healing then continues down the nerve towards the muscle. Recovery time depends on what proportion of the nerve was torn, the size of the gap the new growth needs to traverse, and where along the nerve the rupture is located. These injuries will not be healed in 3 months, but may be healed in 6 months. In most cases, these injuries will lead to secondary and tertiary deformities that will have to be addressed (see Chs. 3-4). It is important to distinguish between preganglionic ruptures and postganglionic ruptures, because they have different healing capabilites. If the cell body of the neuron is injured or disconnected from the nerve, there is no hope of axon regeneration.

Injury to nerves that branch proximally to the brachial plexus roots indicates possible avulsion. These include injuries to the phrenic nerve (C4-C5) which presents as an elevated hemidiaphragm, the long thoracic nerve (C5-C6-C7) which results in winged scapula due to serratus anterior paralysis, and the dorsal scapular nerve (C5) which paralyzes the rhomboid, and the sympathetic chain (C8-T1) which leads to Horner's syndrome. Note that injury to the dorsal scapular nerve, which helps stabilize the position of the scapula, may lead to a significant SHEAR deformity, and this must be looked for in all infants and children with an injury to the brachial plexus. Additionally, injuries to the suprascapular nerve (resulting in absence of rotator cuff function) and the thoracodorsal nerve (resulting in the absence of latissimus dorsi function) can also indicate a proximal injury. If any of these muscle deficits are apparent, confirmation of avulsion should be sought through additional diagnostic testing, and surgical reconstruction of the nerves using nerve transfer techniques may be needed.

In the case of a partial rupture or stretch, it is advisable to wait and see if the nerves are able to heal themselves. The small size of an infant is an advantage in the healing process. Since nerves grow at about 1 inch per month, the average 12 inch span between the injury and the hand can be regenerated in one year. Children also have the advantage of an especially adaptable nervous system. If the healing is delayed, however, muscles will begin to atrophy, and eventually lose the ability to respond to nerve impulses altogether[23]. Often, the healing process creates new nerve paths and connections, or takes advantage of redundant connections. If the brain is not trained to use these connections, muscular co-contractions and other secondary effects may result (see Chs. 2-3). Monitoring recovery can identify these effects early on so that physical therapy and other methods can minimize the occurrence of secondary and tertiary deformities. Learning to use the reformed and rerouted nerve impulses is a priority for therapeutic care during this time.

Clinical Monitoring of Initial Recovery

The most widely-accepted indicator for prognosis following brachial plexus injury in infants is the speed at which antigravity function returns to the biceps muscle. Biceps recovery has proved to be a useful indicator of outcome and a reasonable guide for whether to recommend surgical repair of the brachial plexus[19, 24-27]. In order to understand the reason that the single indicator of biceps recovery can be used to predict outcome, the previously discussed location/pattern and severity/type determinants of brachial plexus injury must be considered. Understanding these concepts will also clarify the recommended timeline for nerve related intervention.

The biceps and deltoid muscles are innervated by nerves originating chiefly in the C5-C6 roots. In the majority of obstetric brachial plexus injuries the injury to C5 is more severe than the other roots (except in cases where the lower roots are avulsed). This means that it typically takes more time to recover muscles innervated by C5 than the other roots. The timeline of biceps and deltoid function recovery is used as an indicator of recovery speed[19, 24].

Biceps function (elbow flexion) is simpler to determine in infants than deltoid function since deltoid strength is often masked by the presence of opposing contractures. Some researchers consider active external rotation and supination, which are also affected by upper root injury, though these can be difficult to assess at 3 months[28]. Studies of brachial plexus recovery commonly quote the age (in months) in which antigravity biceps function is noted. A few studies found that the inclusion of hand and wrist function indicators resulted in improved accuracy of early prognosis[12, 22].

Studies of the natural history of brachial plexus injuries acquired at birth reveal trends roughly linking biceps recovery with prognosis[27, 29]. Recovery of antigravity strength to a child's upper trunk-innervated muscles within the first 2-3 months generally precedes full recovery within the first 1-2 years. The recovery, however, does not always restore normal function. Intermediate groups, with some recovery of biceps function between 3 and 6 months, will develop limited motion and strength. Children without biceps function by 6 to 9 months appear to have the most significant deformities later in life.

No group involved in the treatment of obstetric brachial plexus injuries would suggest that all cases should be treated identically. Several attempts have been made at analyzing the outcomes, so that future patients can be evaluated earlier and treated in the best way possible to maximize the recovery of useful muscle function[19, 22, 24]. Guidelines for when to consider nerve reconstruction by surgical intervention are controversial. A variety of recommendations have been made by surgeons based on their own experiences with patients. Two of the main criteria that have been repeatedly used have been discussed above, i.e., extent of injury and speed of recovery. Narakas's four classes of injury all recover with different speeds, showing that the two main criteria are linked.

Gilbert and others first advocated surgery for children with no biceps function after three months[30, 31]. It is clear that the three month mark does select some patients with poorer recovery, however, a significant number of patients show marked improvement with recovery of biceps function as late as 9 months. Waters, Kline and Noetzel have all advocated waiting at least 6 months[32], if not 9-12[33, 34] before intervening with nerve surgery for infants.

Michelow used indicators of hand and wrist function, in addition to traditional measures of biceps function, at three months to improve 12 month recovery predictions[12]. This system eliminated a significant number of patients from consideration for early neurosurgery. Strömbeck *et al.* demonstrated that children with hand function had more complete improvement of the arm and shoulder[22]. They believe this is because children are more inclined to use their arm when their hand is functioning. This also shows the importance of physical therapy exercises that encourage use of the affected arm and hand.

There are many factors involved in recovery, including nerve healing, development of contractures and co-contraction situations, and dedication to physical therapy. Even when recovery is delayed, children without nerve repair have been shown to do as well as their surgically treated counterparts[35]. Several studies have noted minor or negligible difference between the long-term recovery of children who underwent neuronal repair procedures and those left to recover naturally[22, 35, 36]. However, attempts at studying this systematically have been complicated by small sample size, non-uniform treatment and the wide variety of injury presentations[34]. Therefore, it has not been established whether surgery is indicated in all patients with slow recovery. It is not proven that the post-operative improvements that children experience are better than what they would have experienced from conservative treatment combined with procedures to treat secondary and tertiary effects.

For these reasons, a number of surgeons advocate conservative treatment for birth brachial plexus injuries[12, 22, 35-38], particulary those of Narakas Group 1 and 2. I agree with this philosophy, and believe that nerve reconstruction may be indicated in approximately 10% of patients without anti-gravity biceps by the age of 6 months. As noted previously, EMG testing of the biceps and deltoid will allow a greater degree of confidence in following the conservative route of management, using Botulinum Toxin A (BTX-A) and muscle/bone surgery to achieve good functional outcomes rather than direct nerve repair. This is a safer paradigm for the child's overall health, and the evidence suggests that outcomes are equivalent to major nerve reconstruction at the site of injury.

Adaptability in the regeneration process adds complexity to the clinical evaluation. Even if C5 and C6 roots are avulsed, some function can be provided by neurons originating from the C7 root[39-41]. Whether these pathways exist in all or some newborns and disappear with age or whether they are newly created pathways or, perhaps, a mixture of both, has not yet been established. In adults, this level of rearrangement during healing is not available, making surgery more important at an earlier stage in the recovery process.

Secondary and tertiary effects are a major concern in children with slow recovery. Treatments for contracture and the tertiary effects caused by prolonged contracture are advanced enough to make the advantages of nerve surgery even smaller.

Diagnostics

It is important to know as much as possible about the location and severity of brachial plexus injury before determining treatment. Diagnostic tests should be utilized to provide additional information and confirm clinical findings. Electromyography, a technique in which an electromyogram (EMG) is used to assess the electrophysiological health of a muscle, can help to distinguish nerve rupture

from neurapraxia. An EMG can be used to evaluate motor nerve conduction capability by recording the sum of all the action potentials produced within a set of muscle fibers, a parameter called the compound muscle action potential (CMAP). An EMG at 4-6 weeks also sets a useful baseline with which to track recovery. Electrical improvements measured with a second EMG at 3-4 months, in combination with clinical observations, will allow a more thorough evaluation of recovery.

It is clear that the more severe the injury, the less chance the body has of healing the injury spontaneously. This makes early identification of candidates for nerve reparation surgery more important. Avulsed nerve roots cannot repair themselves, and can be confirmed in most cases by EMG testing of the paraspinal muscles within the first 6-8 weeks of life. The presence of fibrillation potentials in the paraspinal muscles indicates a very proximal injury, unlikely to be reparable directly. The use of magnetic resonance imaging (MRI) and myelography with computed tomography have a reported success rate of up to 84-94% at positively diagnosing avulsion with an ~12% rate of false positives.

My experience with MRI for preoperative assessment of the spinal roots has been unfavorable. EMG testing is the procedure of choice for preoperative evaluation of nerve-muscle integrity. Despite continuing improvements in diagnostic technology, at this time, the final diagnoses must be made during surgery in complex or unclear cases.

If some roots are avulsed, it is likely that additional roots are also severely damaged. The best time for intervention will depend on which roots are avulsed and the extent of recovery evident for nerves stemming from the other roots.

Recovery speed, monitored both by clinical examination and EMG, provides surgeons with useful information about the severity of the nerve injury. Initially, an EMG can be used to distinguish complete ruptures from injuries in-continuity. As the recovery progresses, new EMG studies can indicate whether there are changes in the nerve's ability to conduct. EMG results can enhance the understanding of an injury during the recovery process. A reduced CMAP correlates with a severe injury[35]. As early as 10 days, CMAPs at less than 10% of the unaffected side were correlated with continued weakness at 6 months[42]. Fibrillation potentials, and reduction of interference pattern have also been connected with poor recovery[38].

EMG and nerve conduction velocity (NCV), a technique used to test the speed with which an action potential travels down a nerve, can show improvements in innervation before they manifest as movement[35]. Birch found that EMG results combined with clinical observations helped differentiate between those children who require surgery and those who would fare well with conservative treatment[38].

This is a critical point and emphasizes that knowledge of and attention to the presence of contractures and co-contraction situations must be an integral part of the evaluation process. Loss of shoulder abduction and flexion are mimicked by contractures of the shoulder internal rotators and adductors; apparent loss of elbow flexion is often mimicked by biceps/triceps co-contraction. Both clinical situations are best managed by non-neurosurgical treatment.

Sometimes co-contractions develop that mask the recovered function, emphasizing the need for newly reinnervated muscles to be trained[43]. It is additionally possible that conduction has been regained via a novel pathway that the brain has not learned to control. This, of course, also complicates EMG testing since the stimulation point for a particular muscle group may have changed. One should be mindful of this, and other caveats of the method (small size of target in infants for example) when interpreting EMG results.

Because the results of electromyography examination are sometimes in conflict with the clinical examination, EMG has not been clearly designated as the standard OBPI evaluation tool. If signs of muscle denervation and lack of conduction persist, surgical repair of the nerves can be considered, but only in the context of the clinical observations. Since surgical exploration is desirable only as a last resort, it is important to follow the speed of recovery in as many ways as possible to best estimate nerve health and recovery.

Non-Surgical Interventions

Most commonly, the EMG shows evidence for significant numbers of active motor units while muscle weakness persists in clinical exams. There are several possible explanations for this phenomenon, all of which give hope for the development of improved therapies in the future[39, 41, 44-46]. Luxury innervation and redirected innervations (circuit and central plasticity) both point to the value of considering approaches other than nerve reconstruction in infant injuries.

Whatever the underlying reasons might be for the delay in using newly reinnervated muscles, it is clear that without training, these connections can continue to lay dormant. Development of the brain-muscle connections is necessary for functional use of the newly reinnervated muscles. There

are alternatives to surgery that encourage the use of newly-innervated muscles. This can be achieved through a combination of neurorehabilitative techniques such as physical and occupational therapies, electrostimulation, neuromotor therapy, BTX-A injections and splinting. Among the most promising of these methods is BTX-A treatment, which relaxes neighboring nerve-muscle pathways while the new ones are being learned.

As described in later chapters of this book, these techniques, together with the development of new surgical treatments for secondary muscle and tertiary bone effects, make primary nerve surgery less prudent. In fact, several surgeons trained in the treatment of obstetric brachial plexus palsy are decreasing the number of neurological interventions that they perform[12, 22, 34-37, 47].

Primary Surgical Solutions

There are three primary surgical solutions: neurolysis, neurotization (nerve transfer) and nerve grafting. These may be performed alone or in combination with each other. The choice of which peripheral nerve surgery technique is appropriate is based on which method will maximize and encourage the natural regenerative process of the nerve. This involves balancing two main factors: scar tissue removal and reduction of the gap over which nerves must regenerate. In many cases, the nerve remains in-continuity, and surgery cannot help during the initial stages of healing. In the majority of cases, natural healing processes result in outcomes similar to or better than nerve reconstruction and biceps function is recovered in the first three months. For the remaining cases, paralyses and secondary developmental issues persist and surgical reconstruction of the nerves should be considered and performed as indicated by electrical and clinical evidence.

It should be noted that over the past 30 years, nerve reconstruction has been the primary method of management for obstetric brachial plexus injuries. It is the accumulating weight of evidence over time that is making nerve reconstruction more of a second-line option for the nerve-injured infant. The results of nerve reconstruction are reliable and solid. There is a morbidity, however, attached to the operation itself. I have been referred several cases of iatrogenic phrenic nerve injury caused during nerve grafting surgery, and I am aware of at least 2 infant deaths that have taken place at outside institutions during the course of nerve grafting. When balanced against the very real option of alternative management techniques, nerve repair must be carefully thought out and all other options explored before

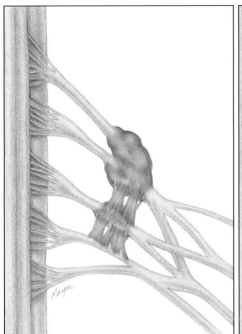

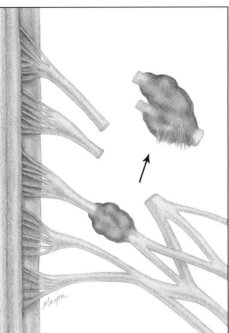

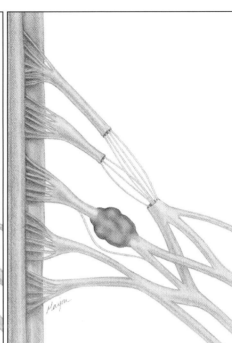

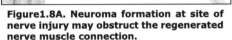

Figure1.8A. Neuroma formation at site of nerve injury may obstruct the regenerated nerve muscle connection.

Figure 1.8B. Resection is performed to remove non-conducting neuromas.

Figure 1.8C. Nerve grafting is used to replace or bypass the gap produced in healthy nerve after resection of the neuroma. Nerve grafting can also be used to repair gaps resulting from ruptures.

being considered as a primary treatment for infants with brachial plexus injury.

In some cases, healing occurs that does not restore the nerve-muscle connection. During healing, new growth may form a neuroma, which is largely scar tissue (Figure 1.8A). Neuromas are also common during healing of ruptures, because of the cloud-like manner in which nerves produce new growth. When some nerve conductivity is maintained through the scar tissue, a neurolysis can be performed to relieve the mechanical obstruction caused by the scarring. It is also possible to remove a nonconducting neuroma (Figure 1.8B) and replace or bypass the gap in healthy nerve with a graft (Figure 1.8C). The diagnosis of a neuroma is difficult, and it is only during surgery that the exact course of injury and healing can be identified. However, surgery of a purely exploratory nature is not recommended. Only after careful clinical monitoring over a six month period, should surgical options be discussed.

Nerve grafting (Figure 1.8C), in which donor nerves from other parts of the body are spliced into the site of nerve rupture, can repair gaps. The sural nerve is commonly used as a donor in these cases. Nerve grafting techniques have improved over the years, and as mentioned, can produce good results.

In the most severe injuries, where avulsion of the nerve root has occurred, surgical intervention is considered much earlier. The natural healing process cannot repair this degree of injury. Since the nerve is torn from the spinal cord, and a connection cannot be made to the original nerve root, neighboring nerves, which can be retrained to stimulate other muscle groups, serve as a signal source after nerve transfer (Figure 1.9). Sources of transfer include the spinal accessory nerves, the intercostal nerves, and other brachial plexus roots and nerves, including transfer from the opposite, uninjured side. Each case is different, and the most desired functions should be considered.

Conclusion

When complete nerve root rupture or avulsion is diagnosed, surgery is considered early on. Self repair is highly unlikely. The individual surgeon will use nerve transfer and grafting, depending on the intra-operative findings and the surgeon's experience. In cases where C8 and T1 are

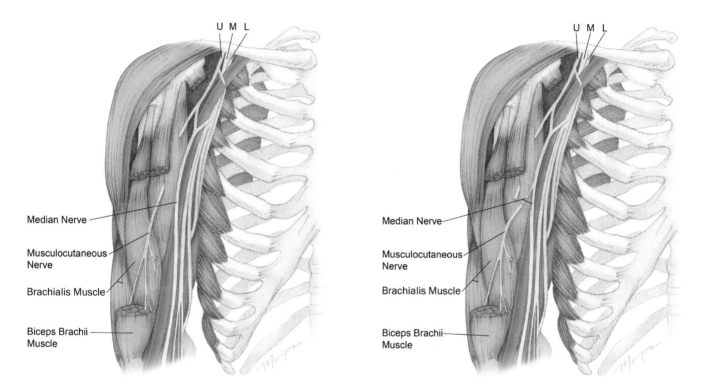

Figure 1.9. In the case of irreparable injury to nerves that supply the biceps brachii and brachialis muscles, transfer of the median nerve is performed. One fascicle group of the median nerve is transferred into the musculocutaneous nerve, distal to the site of injury. The biceps brachii muscle has been partially removed in this illustration. Brachial plexus nerves are indicated in yellow. U, upper trunk; M, middle trunk; L, lower trunk.

involved in addition to C5-C7, hand function is affected, and nerve repair for the upper and middle trunks is more likely to be required. Injuries of C5-C6 do not always warrant operation if injury to C7 is minor.

In most cases the plexus will repair itself more efficiently without surgical help. Within the first three months, range of motion (ROM) exercises performed at each diaper change will encourage motion and maintain flexibility as muscles start regaining power. Physical therapy is important in allowing new movement patterns to be learned, and to maintain range of motion to delay the development of contractures. An initial EMG study is recommended to establish a baseline.

Literature Cited

1. Birch R, Bonney G, Wynn Parry CB. Birth lesions of the brachial plexus. In: Birch R, Bonney G, Wynn Parry CB, eds. In: *Surgical disorders of the peripheral nerves.* New York, NY: Churchill Livingstone; 1998:209-233.

2. Mackinnon SE, Dellon AL. *Surgery of the peripheral nerve.* New York, Stuttgart: Thieme Medical publishers; 1988.

3. Maggi SP, Lowe JB, 3rd, Mackinnon SE. *Pathophysiology of nerve injury.* Clin Plast Surg. Apr 2003;30(2):109-126.

4. Bonnel F. Microscopic anatomy of the adult human brachial plexus: an anatomical and histological basis for microsurgery. *Microsurgery.* 1984;5(3):107-118.

5. Seddon HJ. Three types of nerve injury. *Brain.* 1943;66:237-288.

6. Sunderland S. *Nerves and nerve injuries.* 2 ed. London: Churchill Livingstone; 1978.

7. Mackinnon SE, Dellon AL. Brachial plexus injuries. In: *Surgery of the peripheral nerve.* New York, Stuttgart: Thieme Medical publishers; 1988:423-454.

8. Villavicencio AT, Friedman AH. Surgical management of brachial plexus injuries and thoracic outlet syndrome. In: Grossman RG, Loftus CM, eds. *Principles of neurosurgery.* 2nd ed. Philadelphia: Lippincott-Raven; 1999:679-705.

9. Hardy AE. Birth injuries of the brachial plexus: incidence and prognosis. *J Bone Joint Surg Br.* Feb 1981;63-B(1):98-101.

10. Kay SP. Obstetrical brachial palsy. *Br J Plast Surg.* Jan 1998;51(1):43-50.

11. Levine MG, Holroyde J, Woods JR, Jr., Siddiqi TA, Scott M, Miodovnik M. Birth trauma: incidence and predisposing factors. *Obstet Gynecol.* Jun 1984;63(6):792-795.

12. Michelow BJ, Clarke HM, Curtis CG, et al. The natural history of obstetrical brachial plexus palsy. *Plastic Reconst Surg.* 1994;93(4):675-681.

13. Ubachs, Sloof. Aetiology. In: Gilbert A, ed. *Brachial plexus injuries.* Paris: Martin Dunitz in association with the federation of european societies for surgery of the hand; 2001:151-157.

14. Gilbert A. Obstetrical brachial plexus palsy. In: Tubiana R, ed. *The hand.* Philadelphia, PA: W.B. Saunders Co.; 1993:624-631.

15. Gilbert A, Abbott IR. Long-term evaluation of brachial plexus surgery in obstetrical palsy. *Hand Clinics.* 1995;11(4):583-595.

16. Laurent JP, Lee RT. Birth-related upper brachial plexus injuries in infants: operative and nonoperative approaches. *J Child Neurol.* Apr 1994;9(2):111-117; discussion 118.

17. Al-Qattan MM. Obstetric brachial plexus palsy associated with breech delivery. *Ann Plast Surg.* Sep 2003;51(3):257-264; discussion 265.

18. Slooff AC. Obstetric brachial plexus lesions and their neurosurgical treatment. *Microsurgery.* 1995;16(1):30-34.

19. Narakas AO. Obstetrical Brachial Plexus Injuries. In: Lamb DW, ed. *The paralysed hand.* Vol 2. Edinburgh: Churchill-Livingstone; 1987:116-135.

20. Al-Qattan MM, Clarke HM, Curtis CG. Klumpke's birth palsy. Does it really exist? *J Hand Surg [Br].* Feb 1995;20(1):19-23.

21. Al-Qattan MM. Classification of secondary shoulder deformities in obstetric brachial plexus palsy. *J Hand Surg [Br].* Oct 2003;28(5):483-486.

22. Strömbeck C, Krumlinde-Sundholm L, Forssberg H. Functional outcome at 5 years in children with obstetrical brachial plexus palsy with and without microsurgical reconstruction. *Dev Med Child Neurol.* Mar 2000;42(3):148-157.

23. Sunderland S. *Nerve injuries and their repair : a critical appraisal.* Edinburgh ; New York: Churchill Livingstone; 1991.

24. Gilbert A, Tassin, JL. Obstetric Palsy: Clinical, Pathologic, and Surgical Review. In: Terzis JK, ed. *Microreconstruction of Nerve Injuries.* Philadelphia, PA: WB Saunders; 1987:529-553.

25. Gilbert A, Brockman R, Carlioz H. Surgical treatment of brachial plexus birth palsy. *Clin Orthop Relad Res.* 1991;(264):39-47.

26. Noetzel MJ, Park TS, Robinson S, Kaufman B. Prospective study of recovery following neonatal brachial plexus injury. *J Child Neurol.* Jul 2001;16(7):488-492..

27. Waters PM. Comparison of the natural history, the outcome of microsurgical repair, and the outcome of operative reconstruction in brachial plexus birth palsy. *J Bone Joint Surg Am.* May 1999;81(5):649-659.

28. Hoeksma AF, ter Steeg AM, Nelissen RG, van Ouwerkerk WJ, Lankhorst GJ, de Jong BA. Neurological recovery in obstetric brachial plexus injuries: an historical cohort study. *Dev Med Child Neurol.* Feb 2004;46(2):76-83.

29. McNeely PD, Drake JM. A systematic review of brachial plexus surgery for birth-related brachial plexus injury. *Pediatr Neurosurg.* Feb 2003;38(2):57-62.

30. Gilbert A, Pivato G, Kheiralla T. Long-term results of primary repair of brachial plexus lesions in children. *Microsurgery.* 2006;26(4):334-342.

31. Terzis JK. *Microreconstruction of nerve injuries.* Philadelphia: Saunders; 1987.

32. Noetzel MJ, Wolpaw JR. Emerging concepts in the pathophysiology of recovery from neonatal brachial plexus injury. *Neurology.* Jul 12 2000;55(1):5-6.

33. Kline DG. Perspectives concerning brachial plexus injury and repair. *Neurosurg Clin N Am.* Jan 1991;2(1):151-164.

34. Waters PM. Update on management of pediatric brachial plexus palsy. *J Pediatr Orthop B.* Jul 2005;14(4):233-244.

35. Eng GD, Binder H, Getson P, O'Donnell R. Obstetrical brachial plexus palsy (OBPP) outcome with conservative management. *Muscle Nerve.* Jul 1996;19(7):884-891.

36. Spinner RJ, Kline DG. Surgery for peripheral nerve and brachial plexus injuries or other nerve lesions. *Muscle Nerve.* May 2000;23(5):680-695.

37. Dubuisson A, Kline DG. Indications for peripheral nerve and brachial plexus surgery. *Neurol Clin.* Nov 1992;10(4):935-951.

38. Birch R, Ahad N, Kono H, Smith S. Repair of obstetric brachial plexus palsy: results in 100 children. *J Bone Joint Surg Br.* Aug 2005;87(8):1089-1095.

39. Brown T, Cupido C, Scarfone H, Pape K, Galea V, McComas A. Developmental apraxia arising from neonatal brachial plexus palsy. *Neurology.* Jul 12 2000;55(1):24-30.

40. Korak KJ, Tam SL, Gordon T, Frey M, Aszmann OC. Changes in spinal cord architecture after brachial plexus injury in the newborn. *Brain.* Jul 2004;127(Pt 7):1488-1495.

41. van Dijk JG, Pondaag W, Malessy MJ. Obstetric lesions of the brachial plexus. *Muscle Nerve.* Nov 2001;24(11):1451-1461.

42. Heise CO, Lorenzetti L, Marchese AJ, Gherpelli JL. Motor conduction studies for prognostic assessment of obstetrical plexopathy. *Muscle Nerve.* Oct 2004;30(4):451-455.

43. Pitt M, Vredeveld JW. The role of electromyography in the management of the brachial plexus palsy of the newborn. *Clin Neurophysiol.* Aug 2005;116(8):1756-1761.

44. Vredeveld JW, Blaauw G, Slooff BA, Richards R, Rozeman SC. The findings in paediatric obstetric brachial palsy differ from those in older patients: a suggested explanation. *Dev Med Child Neurol.* Mar 2000;42(3):158-161.

45. Yilmaz K, Caliskan M, Oge E, Aydinli N, Tunaci M, Ozmen M. Clinical assessment, MRI, and EMG in congenital brachial plexus palsy. *Pediatr Neurol.* Oct 1999;21(4):705-710.

46. van Dijk JG, Malessy MJ, Stegeman DF. Why is the electromyogram in obstetric brachial plexus lesions overly optimistic? *Muscle Nerve.* Feb 1998;21(2):260-261.

47. O'Brien DF, Park TS, Noetzel MJ, Weatherly T. Management of birth brachial plexus palsy. *Childs Nerv Syst.* Feb 2006;22(2):103-112.

Chapter 2 Muscle Deformities & Their Management

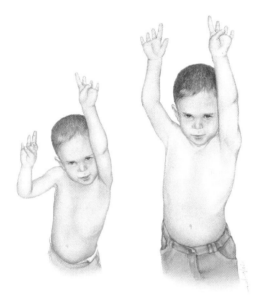

Introduction

The relationship of nerve to muscle is critical to the pathophysiology of obstetric brachial plexus injury in the newborn. The efferent fibers of the cervical nerves stem from the anterior spinal root and merge with the afferent fibers of the posterior spinal root to form the mixed spinal nerves. In the case of the efferent motor neurons, nerve and muscle meet at the neuromuscular junction and, ultimately, each nerve fiber terminates at a voluntary motor fiber. The damage to spinal nerves that occurs in OBPI initially manifests as complete or partial paralysis of the muscles supplied by the damaged nerve fibers.

The most common form of OBPI is Erb's palsy, resulting from injury to the C5-C6 nerves[1]. A pure Erb's palsy is characterized by absence of voluntary abduction and external rotation of the shoulder, elbow flexion and forearm supination, in the presence of relatively intact triceps, forearm and hand function. It is more common to have C5-C6-C7 involvement, although the C7 manifestations are generally milder. Injury to the lower trunk (C8-T1) is typically seen in combination with injury to the upper and middle trunks. A pure Klumpke's paralysis, in which C8-T1 nerves are ruptured or avulsed without middle and upper root involvement, is the most unusual presentation of all OBPI injuries[2].

In my management of obstetric brachial plexus injuries, there has been an evolution toward less aggressive nerve reconstruction with more attention paid to the secondary and tertiary consequences of the initial nerve injury. This is based on developing and quite compelling literature and on my own experience with several thousand patients. The over-riding theme, based on sound scientific data, is always to employ simpler techniques and technology when the choice is available.

I will describe my preferred management for muscle injury as a result of OBPI in this chapter, with supporting clinical and literature evidence.

General Discussion

Neuromuscular Anatomy

The upper and middle trunks of the brachial plexus primarily serve the following upper extremity muscles: rhomboids, serratus anterior, deltoid, subscapularis, supraspinatus, infraspinatus, teres minor, teres major, biceps brachii, brachialis and coracobrachialis (Figure 2.1). Global functions affected by injury to the nerves of the upper and middle trunks include abduction and adduction of the involved extremity, elbow flexion and shoulder rotation (Table 2.I).

The lower arm and hand are primarily innervated by the middle and lower trunks, although there is some involvement of C6 in the median and radial nerves, which are involved with lower arm, wrist and hand function. Functions of the forearm affected by OBPI include supination and pronation of the forearm and wrist, and flexion and extension of the wrist and fingers, among others.

The supraspinatus, infraspinatus, teres minor, and subscapularis muscles surround the glenohumeral (GH) joint

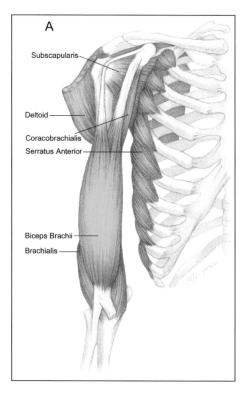

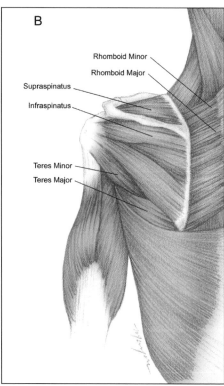

Figure 2.1. Anterior (A) and posterior (B) views of upper extremity and shoulder musculature served by the upper and middle trunks of the brachial plexus.

Table 2.I *Neuromuscular Anatomy*

Muscle	Primary Nerve	Innervation	Movement
Deltoid	C5-C6	axillary	arm flexion/extension, abduction of humerus
Subscapularis	C5-C6	upper & lower subscapular	internal rotation, abduction, flexion of raised arm, stabilizes front of shoulder joint
Supraspinatus	C5-C6	suprascapular	assists deltoid in abduction, support from above
Infraspinatus	C5-C6	suprascapular	rotates head of humerus outward, assist in carrying arm backward, support from behind, adduction
Teres minor	C5	axillary	external rotation and adduction
Teres major	C5-C6	lower subscapular	assist lat in adduction and backward and inward rotation
Latissimus dorsi	C6-C7-C8	long subscapular (thoracodorsal)	depresses and draws back humerus & rotates inward; downward blows
Biceps	C5	musculocutaneous	flexor of the elbow and, to a lesser extent, the shoulder, it is also a powerful supinator
Brachialis	C5 (C6-C7-C8)	musculocutaneous (sometimes radial, too)	elbow flexion
Coracobrachialis	C5	musculocutaneous	elbow flexion, humerus flexion and inward rotation, and at the same time assists in retaining the head of the bone in contact with the glenoid cavity
Triceps brachii	C6-C7-C8	radial	forearm extension, biceps antagonist, assists in humerus extension and adduction

(see Ch. 3 for more on shoulder joint anatomy) and, together with their tendons, form the "rotator cuff". The supraspinatus is located superiorly, the teres minor and infraspinatus are located posteriorly and the subscapularis is located anteriorly to the GH joint. The subscapularis is a strong internal rotator and its tendon forms part of the anterior capsule of the shoulder joint. As such, it is an important contributor to loss of anterior glenohumeral motion in patients with upper brachial plexus injury and resultant muscle imbalances. Along with the deltoid muscle, the muscles of the rotator cuff help to rotate and stabilize the GH joint. The combined downward force created by the infraspinatus, teres minor and subscapularis muscles approximates the upward force exerted by the deltoid. These counteracting forces maintain the humeral head position within the glenoid. The majority of GH rotational force is provided by the supraspinatus, with lesser contributions from the deltoid, subscapularis, infraspinatus and teres minor.

Denervated muscles do not grow at the same rate as their functional, opposing muscles, and muscle imbalances arise. Then, as the nerves heal, muscles regain function in an unbalanced pattern. The strength differences between muscles just regaining their ability to contract and their fully functioning counterparts make it difficult to develop meaningful coordinated function in the newly innervated limb.

The major muscle groups affected by co-contractions are: (1) the shoulder abductors and external rotators (weakened by the C5 injury) versus the adductors and internal rotators of the arm and shoulder (relatively spared in C5 and C6 injuries) and (2) the biceps (weakened by the C6 injury) versus the triceps (relatively spared in C5 and C6 injuries).

The Nath Method

Secondary Deformities Due to OBPI

In most cases of OBPI, significant function of the affected muscles will return, as the regenerative response of the injured nerves is typically brisk. A similar degree of injury in the adult would heal without significant long-term consequences. However, there are critical differences between brachial plexus injury recovery patterns in infants and adults. The most important variable is the rapid growth rate of the affected limb in injured pediatric patients. The second consideration is the asymmetry of injury, upper plexus involvement being more common than middle and lower plexus injury.

The asymmetry of nerve involvement in the face of rapid limb growth leads to secondary muscle imbalances and contractures. Unaffected muscles remain relatively unopposed by denervated muscle groups and lead to adverse effects such as range of motion loss and, in many cases, twisting bony deformities that further decrease function.

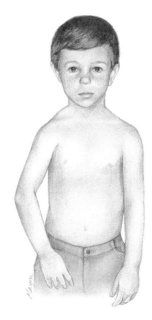

Figure 2.2. Classic arm presentation of OBPI patients with secondary effects to the bone and muscle. Arm is medially rotated and abducted at the shoulder, the forearm is pronated and elbow is flexed.

While the abductor/external rotator and adductor/internal rotator imbalance is generally known as a contracture situation affecting the adductors and internal rotators, it is more accurate to attribute the deformity to both co-contraction and contracture.

In both situations, unopposed contraction of the unaffected muscle group(s) creates a tethering effect that limits passive range of motion of the unbalanced muscles. This leads to the typical arm position seen in children with OBPI: abducted and medially rotated at the shoulder, forearm pronated (the major supinator of the forearm is an intact biceps muscle), and flexed at the elbow (Figure 2.2).

Management of these situations by surgeons has often reflexively been to reconstruct the injured nerves. It is important to keep in mind the background of the surgeons holding the philosophy of aggressive nerve grafting. A recent manuscript detailing the experiences of 22 international surgical specialists, who claim status as experts in management of patients with OBPI, reveals that around 75% treat 15 or fewer patients *per year*, and the top 2 surgeons in the survey (9%) claim a yearly volume of OBPI patients of only about 30 patients[3]. By comparison, Rollnik's group evaluated 482 children, arriving at the conclusion that conservative management was preferable. A growing body of literature, however, suggests that nerve reconstruction should be reserved for only the most severely injured, about 10% or so of the total that are generally evaluated as requiring surgery. My own experience with over 250 patient visits per year leads me to agree with the conservative approach when possible[4].

In Rollnik's study, only 2.5% developed biceps-triceps co-contraction[4]. A far greater number of children, however, will develop significant contractures in the shoulder. Hoeksma *et al*. report that at least one-third of the patients with late (>3 weeks) or incomplete neurological recovery developed contractures of the shoulder[5, 6]. In the same study, 64% of the children with incomplete recovery developed contractures.

The data clearly show that the main issue addressed during treatment of the majority of these children should not be nerve reconstruction, but correction of muscle imbalances and bony deformities that are a consequence of the initial nerve injury.

Muscular imbalances and co-contraction of the limb lead to long-term developmental effects. In addition to impairing the overall function of the involved extremity, an imbalance of muscle strength around the joints will cause skeletal deformities by hindering and/or altering the development of bones, muscles and other soft tissue[5, 7]. The primary effects are tethering of shoulder movement and malpositioning of the arm, each a significant functional problem, but devastating in combination.

The traditional model of OBPI management, primarily presented by Gilbert, holds that full recovery of strength is not expected by those who have not recovered biceps function by the third month[8]. Furthermore, only infants who recover antigravity biceps strength in the first 4-6 weeks of life may have symmetry of their shoulder girdles upon long-term examination[1, 9]. Even these two, and similar other papers, do not discuss the scapular deformity that exists in these patients (the SHEAR deformity, see Chs. 3-4), and probably under-report the true incidence of significant limb and shoulder deformity consequent to any major nerve injury sustained at the time of birth.

Children with even mild persistent neurological deficits at the age of 3 months have a higher risk of long-term upper extremity dysfunction[1, 9]. In a study of 134 infants, 8% developed shoulder abnormality before the age of one year[10]. As a result, surgical interventions such as those mentioned in the previous chapter, including microneurolysis or nerve reconstruction, are recommended by some clinicians[8, 11, 12]. Due to the aggressive nature of this procedure, however, others do not recommend surgical exploration until 9 months of age for upper trunk lesion patients who demonstrate impaired elbow flexion[13].

Assessment

A number of systems are currently employed to assess range of motion in OBPI patients[14]. The two predominant systems were introduced by Mallet[15] and Gilbert[16]. The Modified Mallet System assesses the ability to carry out five movements: abduction, external rotation, hand to back of neck, hand to lower spine and hand to mouth. Each function receives a score of 1 through 5 (1 indicates no function, 5 indicates full function). It must be understood when comparing treatment modalities that the scores of individual patients should not be compared. Active shoulder function is affected by the glenohumeral relationship, shoulder capsule, strength and physical properties of the muscles and the nervous system, therefore, one should compare scores before and after treatment to evaluate the improvement gained by each patient. The Gilbert System classifies degree of shoulder paralysis into six stages based on the abduction and lateral rotation ability (Stage 0 indicates complete paralysis, Stage V indicates abduction >120° with active lateral rotation). I score my results based on the Nath modification of Mallet's system that includes additional functions and positions that I find important (Figure 2.3). My expanded Mallet system incorporates not only static positions (arm at rest) but also includes external rotation and the situation of fixed forearm supination deformity. These functions must be accounted for in any comprehensive evaluation of the OBPI patient.

Treatment

Range of Motion Exercises

Research has shown that immobilization of muscles may be associated with muscle atrophy, range of motion loss, decreased muscle growth in length, loss of tissue mass and an increase in passive elastic stiffness[17]. In addition, changes in the amount and orientation of intramuscular connective tissue also seem to contribute to decreased muscle elasticity[17].

It is critically important for OBPI patients to begin gentle exercises that utilize all of the soft tissues and joints of the affected extremity (Figure 2.4). Infant range of motion exercises strengthen the joints and muscles as well as minimize muscle contractures that can inhibit passive range of motion and cause osseous deformities. However, these exercises should not be limited to physical therapy sessions. Rather, they should be implemented into the patient's daily routine and performed as often as possible (*e.g.*, at diaper change, feeding and bath times). Research supports the idea that functional changes to the muscle can be achieved in the absence of neurological function[18-20]. To maximize effectiveness, parents should demonstrate their technique to their physical therapist monthly. Inappropriate technique can not only minimize benefits, but can also cause additional damage such as radial epiphyseal subluxation[21, 22]. Furthermore, excessive shoulder abduction in the face of axillary and pec-

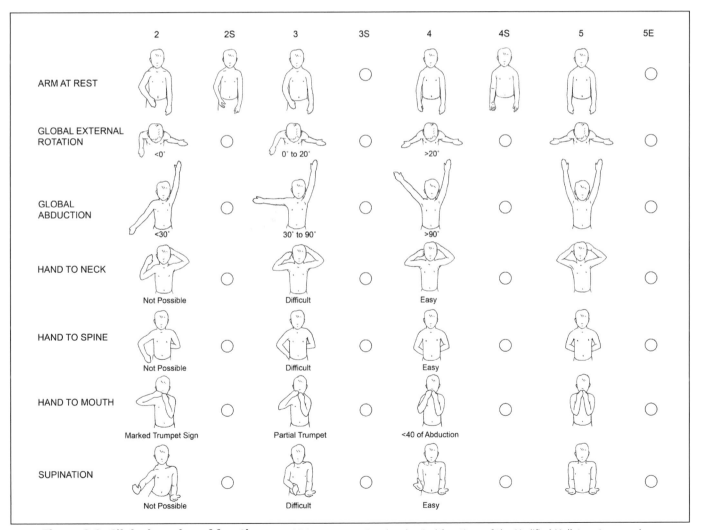

Figure 2.3. Clinical scoring of function. In addition to assessing the classical functions of the Modified Mallet system, supination and the resting position are evaluated. To further define deformity, I score fixed forearm supination (positions 2S, 3S and 4S) as well as external rotation position (5E).

SHOULDER FLEXION

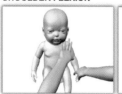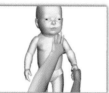

Infant is lying on back. Stabilize shoulder
with one hand and wrist with the other.
Lift the arm up to the level of the shoulder,
thumb leading, elbow straight.

SHOULDER ABDUCTION

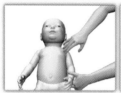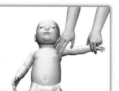

Infant is lying on his/her back. Stablize shoulder
with one hand and forearm with the other.
Lift the arm sideways away from the body,
bring the arm up to the level of the shoulder.

SHOULDER ROTATION

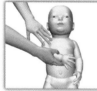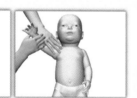

Infant is lying on his/her back. Hold arm at shoulder
with one hand and forearm with the other. Bring
forearm down towards midline with elbow bent,
draw forearm out to side away from body.

WRIST ABDUCTION AND ADDUCTION

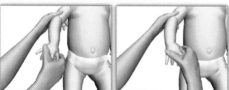

Infant is lying on his/her back. Stabilize forearm
with one hand while holding child's hand with
your other hand. Move wrist from side to side.

ELBOW FLEXION AND EXTENSION

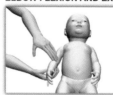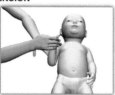

Infant is lying on his/her back.
Stabilize the elbow and hold wrist with other hand.
Bend arm at the elbow, then straighten

FOREARM SUPINATION AND PRONATION

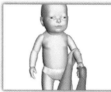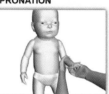

Infant is lying on his/her back. Stabilize upper arm
with one hand by cupping the elbow and
hold the wrist with the other hand.
Roll the forearm and hand up,
then roll the forearm and hand down.

FINGER FLEXION AND EXTENSION

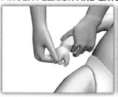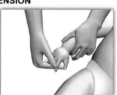

Infant can be lying or sitting.
Stabilize wrist with one hand while
holding child's fingers with the other.
Bend the fingers, then straighten.

FINGER ADDUCTION AND ABDUCTION

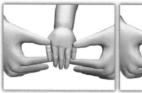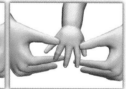

Infant can be lying or sitting. Hold the child's
wrist straight with palm open and fingers
held straight. Spread the fingers apart gently,
then bring them back together.

Figure 2.4. Infant Range of Motion Exercises. To be performed very gently. Each position should be held for 30 seconds
and each motion repeated 10-15 times, only until mild resistance is felt. Exercises should be implemented into daily routine and demonstrated to patient's therapist once a month.

toralis contractures can lead to inferior dislocation of the humeral head, a particularly difficult problem to treat.

Botulinum Toxin A

Botulinum Toxin A (BTX-A) is a neurotoxin that inhibits the release of the neurotransmitter acetylcholine from presynaptic vesicles at the neuromuscular junction, inhibiting the strength of muscle contraction[23]. In recent literature, the use of BTX-A to treat biceps/triceps co-contraction has been supported[4, 24, 25]. Triceps injections have clinically shown good and maintained improvements in biceps movement and strength[26].

Early results show that the benefits of BTX-A are greater the earlier it is used, before abnormal motor patterns are learned[26, 27]. The youngest patients (4 months) showed the greatest increase in shoulder movement after BTX-A treatment for medial rotation[27], although this has not been effective long-term, in my experience. Yet, early intervention with BTX-A may allow infants to develop an awareness of the affected arm that sometimes would not materialize until much later, if at all. This therapy is most effective when combined with intensive occupational/motor learning therapy to teach contracted muscles how to remain relaxed while training newly recovered muscles how to function[26, 27].

Although results for biceps/triceps co-contraction are compelling, BTX-A injections to treat latissimus dorsi, teres major, pectoralis and subscapularis contractures[26] do not seem as effective[26] as triceps injections, probably owing to the larger mass of these muscles.

Surgical Correction

In an effort to treat secondary deformities that arise from OBPI, several corrective methods of soft tissue remodeling

Biceps Tendon *Lengthening*

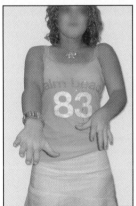
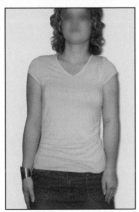

As in other cases of asymmetric nerve injury, muscle imbalances can occur where the biceps is stronger than the opposing triceps muscle. This can occur in a C5-C7 injury where the biceps recovers faster, thereby overpowering the triceps. Typically, serial casting and splinting will not achieve long-term benefits; surgical lengthening of the biceps tendon is an option in these cases.

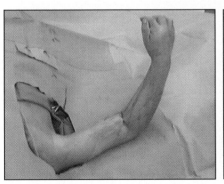
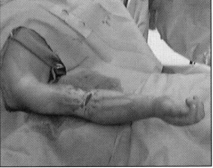

The technique is a Z-lengthening of the tendon from the region of the musculotendinous junction distally. The added length that is achieved allows straightening of the elbow and provides additional length to the arm.

have been developed, including: tendon lengthening, tendon transfer and tendon release procedures (see box on biceps tendon lengthening). Tendon releases are commonly performed surgeries that transfer the insertion point (in bone) of a particular tendon to a new insertion location (either tendon or bone). This allows the action of a strong muscle to be applied in a new way. To date, the most widely used tendon transfers used to treat brachial plexus injuries are adaptations of Sever's original pectoralis major and subscapularis tendon release (Table 2.II)[28].

In a modification introduced by Hoffer and Phipps, contracted internal rotators (latissimus dorsi, teres major and pectoralis major) are released and attached to the point of infraspinatus insertion on the rotator cuff[29]. Improvements in abduction and external rotation are seen in these patients[9, 30, 31]. Various degrees of success have been achieved by others with variations in both the location of the transfer insertion and in the timing of the release in relation to the transfer[32-34].

Compression neuropathy of the axillary nerve has recently been shown to be a contributing factor in cases of persistent muscle weakness. Decompression and neurolysis of the infraclavicular brachial plexus, including the axillary and musculocutaneous nerves has proved helpful to obstetric brachial plexus patients[35].

The Quad Procedure

In my experience, the traditional soft tissue release operations do not adequately address the pathophysiology of the shoulder. However, by coupling neurolysis and decompression of the axillary nerve with an untethering release of soft tissue contractures that limit abduction power, improved shoulder abduction and flexion function in patients with partially recovered brachial plexus injuries is seen. I have modified the combination of muscles released and their inset positions to improve upon a previously described operation by Narakas[36].

Table 2.II *Commonly performed soft tissue procedures*

concomitant release tendon transfer tendon insertion point	Name	Year	n.	Follow-up (yrs)	Improvement in abduction
pectoralis major	Hoffer[39]	1998	8 [6 pts. C5-C6]	2 to 5	~80° passive
LD + TM **infraspinatus**	Phipps & Hoffer[29]	1995	56	5	~46° active
±teres major **LD (± TM)** **supraspinatus**	Pagnotta, Haerle & Gilbert[30]	2004	203 [43 C5-C6 at 6 years]	1, 3, 6, 10, 15	~25° ~60°
± **LD + TM** **infraspinatus**	Waters & Bae[9] Waters & Peljovich[12]	2005 1999	25 32 [10 pts. C5-C6]	3.6 (2 to 10) 1.6 (0.3-5.3)	0.9 pts Mallet† 1.1 pts. Mallet†
±subscapularis **LD + TM** **infraspinatus**	Safoury[31]	2005	32 [18 pts. C5-C6]	2.3 (1.5 to 3.5)	~3 pts Gilbert‡
release of other muscles is staged **LD** **rotator cuff (older),** **humeral head (younger)**	Al_Qattan[37]	2003	12	4 (3 to 5)	~40° active
±subscapularis **LD + TM** **infraspinatus**	Aydin, Ozkan & Onel[38]	2004	46 (older children) [12 pts. C5-C6]	3.4 (2 to 5)	~30°
Quad Procedure **subscapularis, pectoralis major and minor** **LD + TM** **teres minor**	**Nath**[43]	**2007**	**72**	**5.1 (2 to 8)**	**~117° active**

Table Legend
LD: latissimus dorsi, TM: teres major
±: as deemed appropriate
†: abduction according to Mallet: 2: <30°, 3: 30° - 90°, 4: >90°
‡: abduction according to Gilbert: 1: =45°, 2: <90°, 3: =90°, 4: <120°, 5: >120°, 6: >150°

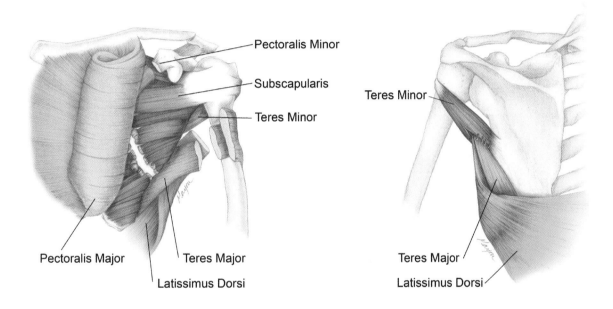

SURGICAL RELEASE OF:
Pectoralis Minor, Pectoralis Major,
Teres Major, Latissimus Dorsi,
and partial release of the Subscapularis

REATTACHMENT OF:
Teres Major and Latissimus Dorsi
to Teres Minor

Pectoralis Minor

Subscapularis

Teres Minor

Pectoralis Major

Teres Major

Latissimus Dorsi

Teres Minor

Teres Major

Latissimus Dorsi

Figure 2.5. The Mod Quad Procedure improves shoulder abduction and flexion. Left, release of major internal rotator muscles: subscapularis (not shown), teres major, latissimus dorsi, pectoralis major and minor. Right, teres major and latissimus dorsi are transferred to the teres minor, increasing external rotation, abduction and scapular stability. Neurolysis and decompression of the axillary nerve further increase range of motion.

My procedure is referred to as the "Quad" surgery (Figure 2.5) because it is based on the following four steps:

(1) Latissimus dorsi muscle release and transfer for external rotation and abduction.

(2) Teres major muscle release and transfer for scapular stabilization.

(3) Subscapularis release without transfer.

(4) Axillary nerve decompression and neurolysis.

Depending on the individual child, other nerve decompressions or muscle/tendon transfers (such as pectoralis muscle releases) might be performed at the same time (the modified Quad or "Mod Quad" procedure).

In the Mod Quad procedure, the latissimus dorsi, teres major, subscapularis and pectoralis muscle contractures are released. The latissimus dorsi and teres major muscles are sutured to a low position in the teres minor muscle, as performed by Narakas[36]. This enhances the stabilizing effect of the rotator cuff, enabling the deltoid to act more effectively while not tethering shoulder abduction and flexion ability. Inherent to this procedure is an understanding that the presence of anti-gravity deltoid strength is masked by antagonistic muscle contractures in the axilla and chest.

Previously described surgical techniques have improved external rotation by inserting the tendons higher in the shoulder and more laterally than the Quad surgery (Table 2.II)[9, 12, 29-31, 37-39]. This methodology improves external rotation, but actively inhibits abduction and flexion. The Nath Method corrects external rotation and supination defects in separate procedures of the shoulder girdle bones (the SHEAR deformity, see Chs. 3-4) and aims to achieve maximum shoulder abduction and flexion with the Quad surgery.

Recently, axillary nerve impingement has been confirmed to be a separate and common reason for shoulder impairment in children with brachial plexus injury[35]. Axillary nerve decompression and neurolysis due to secondary compression of the axillary nerve within the quadrangular space has been an intrinsic component of the soft tissue Quad procedure, described above, since the surgery's inception in 1996. The pathophysiology is related to inferior subluxation of the humeral head, secondary to deltoid weakness, as a result of the C5 injury.

The anatomic course of the axillary nerve carries it between the humeral head and the superomedial border of the triceps fascia of the quadrangular space before it innervates the deltoid. This position makes it susceptible to compression by the displaced humeral head, inhibiting nerve conductivity. A vicious cycle initiates as the compromised axillary nerve further weakens the deltoid, allowing more subluxation of the humeral head against the axillary nerve until stability is finally reached at a level that is unfavorable with respect to shoulder function. As part of the Quad procedure, I routinely perform decompression of the axillary nerve and further address the periarticular compression by releasing the fascia of the long head of the triceps muscle.

Some surgeons perform the muscle release and transfer procedures in stages[1, 9, 31, 39-41]. Theoretically, this allows for improvement in passive external rotation of the shoulder prior to muscle transfer. My approach bears a closer resemblance to Hoffer and Phipps' surgery[1, 9, 31, 39] in which the latissimus dorsi and pectoralis major insertion transfers are performed concomitant to the muscle release. While Hoffer and Phipps transfer the insertions to the rotator cuff, I suture the transferred muscles closer to the origin of the teres minor, ensuring full passive abduction of the arm. This is similar to the technique employed by Narakas[42]. The rationale for doing this is that re-inserting the already contracted muscles high to the rotator cuff or humerus would further tether the joint.

My method makes it possible for the weakened abductors to perform antigravity movements untethered by the stronger muscles which have been released. I also routinely include the axillary nerve decompression that has been previously described[35]. The long-term effects of restored shoulder abduction by the Quad procedure was assessed in 72 obstetric brachial plexus patients with paralysis (Narakas Groups 2, 3 and 4) that did not resolve by the first six months of age. Patients presented with at least partially recovered C5-C6 brachial plexus injuries and significant loss of abduction ability with easily palpable contractures of the pro-gravity muscles, i.e., latissimus dorsi, teres major and pectoralis major. All patients had preoperative abduction values of less than 90° (mean: 41°). Clinical evidence of at least limited active deltoid abduction and flexion ability was required in order to be eligible for the Quad procedure. Patients whose shoulder elevation merely consisted of shrugging movements with little humeral rotation away from the trunk and who did not exhibit clear contraction of the intact adductors and internal rotator muscles were not eligible for the surgical procedure. Patients with significant bony abnormalities such as scapular elevation and humeral head subluxation were not excluded because these abnormalities are believed to be more related to the medial rotation deformity and not a cause of the abduction loss.

In this series of patients and several thousand others on whom I have operated, there has routinely been an impressive improvement in active shoulder abduction (Figure 2.6). 53 of the 72 children (74%) who underwent this procedure began at a lower functional status for abduction than in other similar studies and had resultant active abduction of 160° or more. This would not have been possible if the released muscles had been inserted to the rotator cuff. My results in active shoulder abduction correction are superior to those achieved in previous reports (Table 2.II)[9, 12, 29-31, 37-39]. These results are based on a follow-up time greater than all but one of those studies. While there often was some improvement of external rotation and supination in this series of patients, these are more related to osseous derangements (the SHEAR deformity) and definitive reconstruction will require corrective bone surgery.

Timing of the Quad surgery is based on the presence of muscle tightness of the shoulder internal rotators and adductors, regardless of age. As developmental shoulder deformities are being recognized at earlier ages in this population, there has been a trend toward earlier soft-tissue surgery. Hoffer and Phipps[39] and Pearl et al.[40], have recommended waiting until the child is three years of age when no further spontaneous recovery is expected. On the other hand, in addition to the beneficial effects on active movement and function, tendon release and relocation minimizes the progression of glenoid retroversion and GHJ instability (see Chs. 3 and 4)[9]. It has already been shown that posterior shoulder subluxation is seen by 3 months of age[10]. For these reasons, I do not advocate delaying the release of tight, unbalanced muscle groups once they are diagnosed.

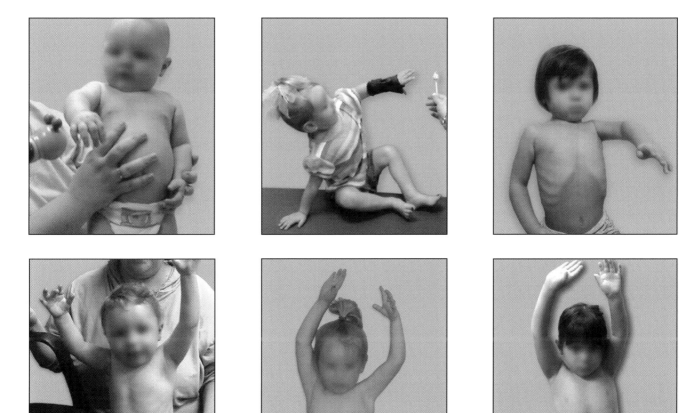

Figure 2.6. Patients demonstrate improved abduction and overhead range of motion after Mod Quad surgery. Three OBPI patients with limited abduction before Mod Quad surgery (top row) show dramatic increases in overhead range of motion after the procedure (bottom row).

Surgical Procedure

Patients are given general anesthesia. Incisions are created in the axilla. Upon identification of the latissimus dorsi, dissection of the muscle proceeds medially across the latissimus dorsi into the subscapularis fossa. The subscapularis muscle is lengthened in a medial to lateral direction using electrocautery. Dissection proceeds down to the periosteum of the medial scapular face.

The tendon of the latissimus dorsi is dissected superiorly. At the superior extent of the dissection, the latissimus tendon is retracted laterally, exposing the underlying tendon of the triceps (long head). The tendon of the latissimus dorsi is detached sharply from its insertion into the humerus. Anterior to the latissimus dorsi tendon, the teres major tendon is separately released. Both tendons are now dissected towards the inferior part of the scapula. This exposes the triceps as well as its superomedial border.

At the superomedial border of the triceps origin, the axillary nerve is routinely noted to be compressed by a combination of humeral head inferior subluxation (due to deltoid weakness subsequent to the original C5 injury) and the dense fascia of the triceps in the quadrangular space. The triceps fascia is released sharply, thereby decompressing the axillary nerve. A full internal neurolysis is performed to remove epineurial scar tissue. Direct electrical stimulation of the axillary nerve is used to confirm improved active movement of the deltoid muscle following neurolysis.

An incision is created in the anterior axillary fold, and the pectoralis major tendon is identified. The distal muscle fibers and tendon of the pectoralis muscle are sharply released with electrocautery. Sufficient lengthening, as determined during surgery, is performed to allow additional passive range of external rotation. The underlying tendon of the pectoralis minor is released sharply under direct vision.

Following release of the pectoralis major and minor tendons, a blunt release of the connective tissue of the anterior glenohumeral joint capsule may be performed through the axillary incision, to allow improved anterior movement of the humeral head within the joint. A formal subscapularis tendon lengthening and anterior capsule release is not generally performed at this time, but may be done if needed. With the arm placed in full abduction and external rotation, the tendons of the latissimus dorsi and teres major are individually sutured into the teres minor.

The wound is closed in two layers with absorbable sutures over a drain. Postoperative care includes immobilization in an abduction "Statue of Liberty" splint (Figure 2.7) for four to six weeks. During the next six weeks, the splint is worn only at night. Full shoulder movement is permitted after the initial four week postoperative period but no weight-bear-

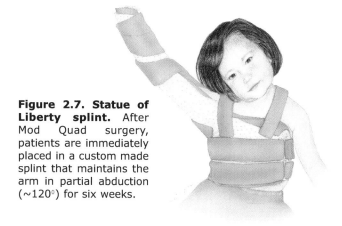

Figure 2.7. Statue of Liberty splint. After Mod Quad surgery, patients are immediately placed in a custom made splint that maintains the arm in partial abduction (~120°) for six weeks.

ing or strengthening is allowed for an additional several weeks depending on the original severity of the injury and intraoperative factors. Rapid improvement in measured shoulder abduction is generally expected. Physical therapy is prescribed three times a week for at least 3 months and swimming is encouraged to prevent stiffness.

Literature Cited

1. Waters PM. Update on management of pediatric brachial plexus palsy. *J Pediatr Orthop B.* Jul 2005;14(4):233-244.
2. Narakas AO. Obstetrical brachial plexus injuries. In: Lamb DW, ed. *The paralysed hand.* Vol 2. Edinburgh: Churchill-Livingstone; 1987:116-135.
3. Shah AK, Zurakowski D, Jessel RH, Kuo A, Waters PM. Measuring surgeons' treatment preferences and satisfaction with nerve reconstruction techniques for children with unique brachial plexus birth palsies. *Plast Reconstr Surg.* Sep 15 2006;118(4):967-975.
4. Rollnik JD, Hierner R, Schubert M, et al. Botulinum toxin treatment of cocontractions after birth-related brachial plexus lesions. *Neurology.* Jul 12 2000;55(1):112-114.
5. Hoeksma AF, Ter Steeg AM, Dijkstra P, Nelissen RG, Beelen A, de Jong BA. Shoulder contracture and osseous deformity in obstetrical brachial plexus injuries. *J Bone Joint Surg Am.* Feb 2003;85-A(2):316-322.
6. Hoeksma AF, Wolf H, Oei SL. Obstetrical brachial plexus injuries: incidence, natural course and shoulder contracture. *Clin Rehabil.* Oct 2000;14(5):523-526.
7. Pearl ML, Edgerton BW. Glenoid deformity secondary to brachial plexus birth palsy. *J Bone Joint Surg Am.* May 1998;80(5):659-667.
8. Gilbert A, Tassin JL. [Surgical repair of the brachial plexus in obstetric paralysis]. *Chirurgie.* 1984;110(1):70-75.
9. Waters PM, Bae DS. Effect of tendon transfers and extra-articular soft-tissue balancing on glenohumeral development in brachial plexus birth palsy. *J Bone Joint Surg Am.* Feb 2005;87(2):320-325.
10. Moukoko D, Ezaki M, Wilkes D, Carter P. Posterior shoulder dislocation in infants with neonatal brachial plexus palsy. *J Bone Joint Surg Am.* Apr 2004;86-A(4):787-793.
11. Birch R, Ahad N, Kono H, Smith S. Repair of obstetric brachial plexus palsy: results in 100 children. *J Bone Joint Surg Br.* Aug 2005;87(8):1089-1095.
12. Waters PM, Peljovich AE. Shoulder reconstruction in patients with chronic brachial plexus birth palsy. A case control study. *Clin Orthop Relat Res.* Jul 1999;(364):144-152.
13. Clarke H, Curtis C. Examination and Prognosis. In: Gilbert A, ed. *Brachial plexus injuries.* London: Martin Dunitz Ltd.; 2001:159-172.
14. Bae DS, Waters PM, Zurakowski D. Reliability of three classification systems measuring active motion in brachial plexus birth palsy. *J Bone Joint Surg Am.* Sep 2003;85-A(9):1733-1738.
15. Mallet J. [Obstetrical paralysis of the brachial plexus. II. Therapeutics. Treatment of sequelae. Priority for the treatment of the shoulder. Method for the expression of results]. *Rev Chir Orthop Reparatrice Appar Mot.* 1972;58:Suppl 1:166-168.
16. Gilbert A. Obstetrical brachial plexus palsy. In: Tubiana R, ed. *The hand.* Philadelphia, PA: W.B. Saunders Co.; 1993:624-631.
17. Gajdosik RL. Passive extensibility of skeletal muscle: review of the literature with clinical implications. *Clin Biomech (Bristol, Avon).* Feb 2001;16(2):87-101.
18. Mills VM. Electromyographic results of inhibitory splinting. *Phys Ther.* Feb 1984;64(2):190-193.
19. Reimers J. Functional changes in the antagonists after lengthening the agonists in cerebral palsy. II. Quadriceps strength before and after distal hamstring lengthening. *Clin Orthop Relat Res.* Apr 1990(253):35-37.
20. Reimers J. Functional changes in the antagonists after lengthening the agonists in cerebral palsy. I. Triceps surae lengthening. *Clin Orthop Relat Res.* Apr 1990(253):30-34.
21. Birch R, Bonney G, Wynn Parry CB. Birth lesions of the brachial plexus. In: Birch R, Bonney G, Wynn Parry CB, eds. *Surgical disorders of the peripheral nerves.* New York, NY: Churchill Livingstone; 1998:209-233.
22. Eng GD, Binder H, Getson P, O'Donnell R. Obstetrical brachial plexus palsy (OBPP) outcome with conservative management. *Muscle Nerve.* Jul 1996;19(7):884-891.
23. Aoki KR, Guyer B. Botulinum toxin type A and other botulinum toxin serotypes: a comparative review of biochemical and pharmacological actions. *Eur J Neurol.* Nov 2001;8 Suppl 5:21-29.
24. Basciani M, Intiso D. Botulinum toxin type-A and plaster cast treatment in children with upper brachial plexus palsy. *Pediatr Rehabil.* Apr-Jun 2006;9(2):165-170.
25. Heise CO, Lorenzetti L, Marchese AJ, Gherpelli JL. Motor conduction studies for prognostic assessment of obstetrical plexopathy. *Muscle Nerve.* Oct 2004;30(4):451-455.

26. DeMatteo C, Bain JR, Galea V, Gjertsen D. Botulinum toxin as an adjunct to motor learning therapy and surgery for obstetrical brachial plexus injury. *Dev Med Child Neurol.* Apr 2006;48(4):245-252.

27. Desiato MT, Risina B. The role of botulinum toxin in the neuro-rehabilitation of young patients with brachial plexus birth palsy. *Pediatr Rehabil.* Jan-Mar 2001;4(1):29-36.

28. Sever JW. Obstetric paralysis: Its etiology, pathology, clinical aspects and treatment, with a report of four hundred and seventy cases. *Am J Dis Child.* December 1916;12(6):541-578.

29. Phipps GJ, Hoffer MM. Latissimus dorsi and teres major transfer to rotator cuff for Erb's palsy. *J Shoulder Elbow Surg.* Mar-Apr 1995;4(2):124-129.

30. Pagnotta A, Haerle M, Gilbert A. Long-term results on abduction and external rotation of the shoulder after latissimus dorsi transfer for sequelae of obstetric palsy. *Clin Orthop Relat Res.* Sep 2004(426):199-205.

31. Safoury Y. Muscle transfer for shoulder reconstruction in obstetrical brachial plexus lesions. *Handchir Mikrochir Plast Chir.* Oct 2005;37(5):332-336.

32. Kirkos JM, Kyrkos MJ, Kapetanos GA, Haritidis JH. Brachial plexus palsy secondary to birth injuries. *J Bone Joint Surg Br.* Feb 2005;87(2):231-235.

33. Ross A, Birch R. Reconstruction of the paralyzed shoulder after brachial plexus injuries. In: Tubiana R, ed. *The hand.* Vol IV. Philadelphia, PA: W.B. Saunders; 1991:126-133.

34. Zancolli E, Zancolli E. Palliative surgical procedures in sequellae of obstetrical palsy. In: Tubiana R, ed. *The hand.* Vol IV. Philadelphia, PA: W.B. Saunders; 1991:602-623.

35. Adelson PD, Nystrom NA, Sclabassi R. Entrapment neuropathy contributing to dysfunction after birth brachial plexus injuries. *J Pediatr Orthop.* Sep-Oct 2005;25(5):592-597.

36. Narakas AO. Muscle transpositions in the shoulder and upper arm for sequelae of brachial plexus palsy. *Clin Neurol Neurosurg.* 1993;95 Suppl:S89-91.

37. Al-Qattan MM. Latissimus dorsi transfer for external rotation weakness of the shoulder in obstetric brachial plexus palsy. *J Hand Surg [Br].* Oct 2003;28(5):487-490.

38. Aydin A, Ozkan T, Onel D. Does preoperative abduction value affect functional outcome of combined muscle transfer and release procedures in obstetrical palsy patients with shoulder involvement? *BMC Musculoskelet Disord.* Aug 3 2004;5:25.

39. Hoffer MM, Phipps GJ. Closed reduction and tendon transfer for treatment of dislocation of the glenohumeral joint secondary to brachial plexus birth palsy. *J Bone Joint Surg Am.* Jul 1998;80(7):997-1001.

40. Pearl ML, Edgerton BW, Kazimiroff PA, Burchette RJ, Wong K. Arthroscopic release and latissimus dorsi transfer for shoulder internal rotation contractures and glenohumeral deformity secondary to brachial plexus birth palsy. *J Bone Joint Surg Am.* Mar 2006;88(3):564-574.

41. Price AE, Grossman JA. A management approach for secondary shoulder and forearm deformities following obstetrical brachial plexus injury. *Hand Clin.* Nov 1995;11(4):607-617.

42. Egloff DV, Raffoul W, Bonnard C, Stalder J. Palliative surgical procedures to restore shoulder function in obstetric brachial palsy. Critical analysis of Narakas' series. *Hand Clin.* Nov 1995;11(4):597-606.

43. Nath RK, Paizi M. Long term results on abduction of the shoulder after reconstructive soft-tissue procedures in obstetric brachial plexus palsy. *J Bone Joint Surg Br.* May 2007;89-B(5):in press.

Chapter 3 Bone Deformities & Their Management

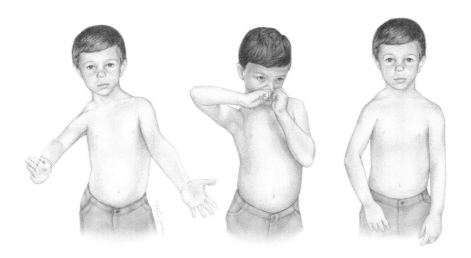

Introduction

Shoulder problems that normally present as weakness of the deltoid and external shoulder rotators (innervated by C5) are the most consistent functional and anatomic derangements that occur in OBPI as a result of significant C5 injury. Long standing muscular imbalances around the shoulder lead to progressive glenohumeral dysplasia and instability[1].

The asymmetric injury clinically presents with muscle tightness in both the internal rotators and adductors of the shoulder. These secondary effects occur since innervation to these muscles is generally less affected by initial nerve injury patterns. As a result, these muscles become overactive in the absence of antagonistic muscle function. Muscle imbalances around the shoulder joint produce atypical musculoskeletal dynamics that alter the growth of the limb. Bony deformities develop as a result of reduced innervation to affected bones[2,3,4,5] and the previously mentioned asymmetric muscle action on developing bony elements of the shoulder. The underlying bony problem is the SHEAR deformity.

General Discussion

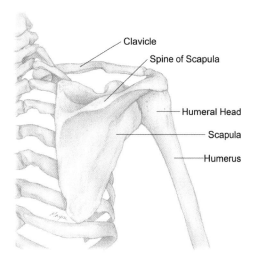

Figure 3.1. Posterior view of right shoulder girdle showing the three primary components: scapula, spine of scapula, humeral head, and clavicle. Humerus is also indicated.

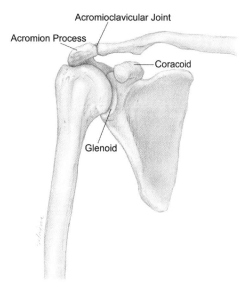

Figure 3.2. Anterior view of the right glenohumeral joint. Acromion process, acromioclavicular joint, and coracoid are indicated in the figure.

Anatomy of the Shoulder Girdle

The primary bones that constitute the shoulder girdle are: the scapula, the clavicle and the humeral head (Figure 3.1). The superior lateral surface of the scapula forms a hollow called the glenoid fossa. The glenoid fossa is also referred to as the glenoid. The humeral head fits into the glenoid to form the ball-and-socket glenohumeral joint (GHJ) (Figure 3.2). The spine of the scapula rises laterally and forms the acromion process posteriorly. The coracoid process protrudes anteriorly.

The clavicle, which is attached at its medial end to the sternum via the sternoclavicular joint (SCJ), is distally attached to the superior surface of the scapula via the acromioclavicular joint (ACJ). The distal acromioclavicular triangle (ACT) has a central role in the typical medial rotation contracture (MRC) deformity seen in OBPI. The anterior surface of the scapula rests on the thorax at an articulation referred to as the scapulothoracic joint (STJ). In actuality, the STJ is not a true "joint", but represents the surface on which the scapula moves in relation to the thorax. Movements of the STJ, ACJ and SCJ are intimately associated because, collectively, they link the bones of the thorax, scapula, clavicle and sternum. Scapular movement results in movement of the ACJ and/or SCJ and, therefore, depends on their integrity.

The GHJ is characterized by a broad range of motion. The surfaces of the GHJ (the humeral head and glenoid fossa) are protected by articular cartilage which also serves to improve congruence of the joint. Further cushioning is supplied by the labrum, a ring of fibrous connective tissue that surrounds the glenoid. A large, dynamic capsule, reinforced by glenohumeral (GH) ligaments and associated muscles, surrounds the entire GHJ.

Although the shoulder joint has unlimited range of motion, in terms of pathophysiology, it can be thought of as having gradations of vertical and horizontal movements that combine to give total range of motion. Pathologic inhibition of vertical movement is due to contractures of the internal rotator and adductor muscles, while deficits in the horizontal plane (loss of external rotation and supination) are due to the bony abnormalities associated with the SHEAR deformity.

The shoulder is under dynamic stabilization forces. That is to say, it is not held in place by any one, fixed anatomical fixture. Rather, the bones, joints and soft tissues of the shoulder function interdependently to hold the shoulder in place while maximizing range of motion. Disruption to this dynamic stabilization, a predictable sequela of OBPI, initiates a chain of destabilizing events within the shoulder.

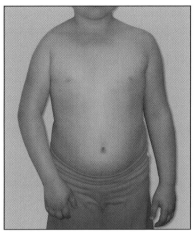

Figure 3.3. Six-year old with right OBPI. Notice deep anterior fold of right axilla as compared with the normal left side. The resting arm position is abducted with flexion of the elbow.

The Nath Method

Tertiary Osseous Deformities Due to OBPI

Advanced bone and muscle abnormalities result in a classic clinical presentation of the extremity at rest (Figure 3.3). There is apparent shortening of the humeral segment of the arm with deeper anterior and posterior axillary folds reflecting the tightness of the underlying latissimus dorsi, teres major and pectoralis muscles and the posterior projection of the humeral head[6]. The medially rotated arm is abducted several degrees, and the elbow consequently flexes. Typically, the dorsum of the hand is visible anteriorly. During active motion of the extremity, abduction is diminished because of the axillary and pectoral muscle tightness. Asymmetry of the shoulder girdle is apparent. Range of passive and active external rotation decreases due to alteration of shoulder dynamics and muscular contractures of the adductor muscles. In severe cases, the occurrence of humeral and forearm bone shortening is not uncommon (see box on Ilizarov bone lengthening).

Humeral Head Subluxation

In some cases, muscular imbalances, that result from partial muscular reinnervation subsequent to OBPI, influence articular surfaces of the shoulder that are particularly susceptible to remodeling. In children, this is confounded by the fact that these forces are taking place in a highly plastic,

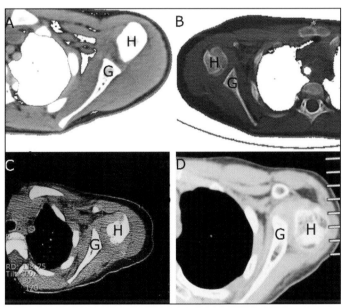

Figure 3.4. Axial CT images demonstrating progression of glenohumeral deformity. A. Normal concentric glenohumeral joint. Glenoid (G) is congruent with humeral head (H). B. Apparent flattening and retroversion of right glenoid. C. Progressed retroversion. D. Severe left glenohumeral joint deformity. Notice humeral head subluxation and advanced glenoid retroversion.

ossifying environment. Collectively, this leads to progressive GHJ deformity. Morphological changes to the glenoid have been well-documented in the literature[1, 7-12]. Advances in imaging technology have greatly improved the characterization and identification of these deformities (Figure 3.4). The early stages of glenoid remodeling are characterized by flattening of the posterior aspect of the glenoid, eventually

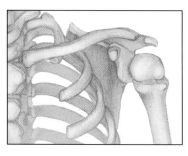

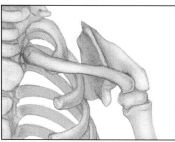

Figure 3.5. Anterior view of normal shoulder girdle (top) and shoulder with SHEAR deformity (bottom). Notice the hypoplasia of the scapula and abnormal position of the acromioclavicular triangle in relation to the humeral head.

leading to the formation of a biconcave glenoid in which the humeral head articulates with the posterior concavity. Some studies report that with the progression of deformity, a pseudoglenoid forms; the posterior concavity becomes distinct and separate from the original anterior glenoid concavity[12]. Progressive subluxation of the humeral head often accompanies changes to the glenoid. The type and severity of deformity is associated with both age and degree of medial rotation contracture.

Scapular Hypoplasia, Elevation and Rotation (SHEAR)

Much consideration has been given in the literature to GHJ deformities that result from OBPI, particularly shoulder dislocation. However, there is a major underlying bony deformity, the SHEAR (Scapular Hypoplasia, Elevation and Rotation) deformity, which has been overlooked. SHEAR essentially consists of abnormal lateral and superior rotation of the scapula (Figure 3.5). This movement deforms the clavicle in a complex manner: the scapular elevation rotates the superior surface of the distal third of the clavicle anteriorly and the lateral scapular migration bends the entire distal third forward. Since the medial end of the clavicle is fixed to the sternum, compensatory movements in response to scapula motion is limited, hence the distal ACT is tilted superiorly, its anterior surface facing more anteriorly. Abnormal morphology of the coracoid, acromion, clavicle and ligaments of the ACT have been reported elsewhere[1, 13]. It has been my experience and the experience of others[13, 14] that these types of deformities progress with age despite ongoing physical therapy.

Ilizarov Bone *Lengthening*

The patient is a 13-year old boy with a complete left brachial plexus injury. He has undergone multiple surgeries including a free functional muscle transfer to the forearm to allow finger movement. He was left with severe bony rotational and shortening deformities that were functionally limiting. In such severe cases, the use of Ilizarov bone distraction technique is appropriate. In this patient, the Ilizarov technique was used for rotation and lengthening of the humerus as well as the forearm. Functional gains are significant as the hand is placed into a more useful position.

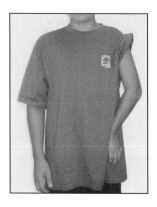
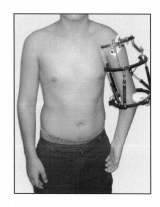
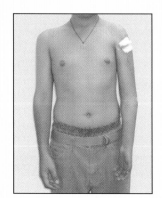
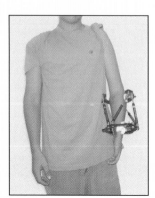

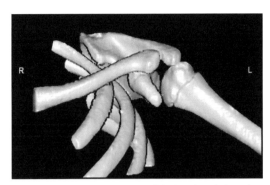

Figure 3.6. 3D-CT of shoulder with SHEAR deformity. The constant downward pressure exerted by the acromion on the humeral head causes the abducted resting position of the arm.

The SHEAR deformity contributes to the characteristic arm position which limits hand-to-mouth function and apparent supination. External rotation of the arm and shoulder is restricted because the ACT impinges against the humeral head. The resulting downward pressure on the humeral head is the anatomic basis for the medial rotation (Figure 3.6). Additionally, there are varying degrees of elbow flaring upon flexion of the elbow (trumpeter's position) and difficulty in placing the hands to the nape of the neck. It is important to understand that muscle and bone deformities are linear consequences of the initial nerve injury occurring during a time of rapid development.

Without the acromion in its usual location stabilizing the GHJ, posterior and inferior subluxation of the humeral head may result. Other tertiary effects include medial humeral rotation, flattening of the glenoid fossa and hooking of the acromion process which may cause further impingement upon the humeral head[1].

It is clear that these anatomic derangements are a potential source of functional loss and progressive disability with loss of quality of life. Patients with untreated OBPI complications report severely impaired function associated with pain during movement. Most of the bony architecture of the shoulder girdle is significantly altered. This fact must be appreciated in order to comprehend the severity of the injury. Successful management of the bony changes in the shoulder will have an important impact on long-term preservation of global function in OBPI patients.

Clinical Evaluation of SHEAR

Physical examination reveals the presence of SHEAR deformity, which is confirmed by 3D-CT (Figure 3.7) whenever possible. Patients' shoulder function is assessed preoperatively and postoperatively by evaluating video recordings of standardized movements following the Nath

Arm Rotated Medially *with Supination (ARMS)*

A frequent and previously under-recognized variant of the medial rotation contracture is the concurrent presence of a fixed supination deformity along with the humeral medial rotation deformity (the ARMS deformity). The sequence is recognized clinically by the parallel positioning of the volar surface of the forearm to the anterior surface of the arm. The usual association between these entities is that the forearm volar surface is perpendicular or over-pronated in relation to the anterior arm surface.

The clinical importance is that the excessive medial rotation of the arm is camouflaged by the excessive forearm supination at the level of the hand. Therefore, to the untrained eye, the hand is in the neutral position and symmetric with the uninjured side. However, observation of the elbow crease shows that it is indeed not visible anteriorly and further observation notes the abnormal relationship between the volar forearm and anterior arm surfaces.

Correction requires surgery for both the humeral and forearm bony deformities.

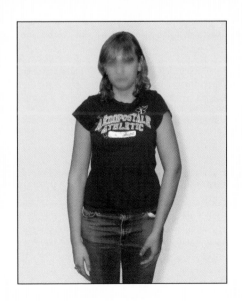

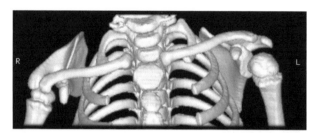

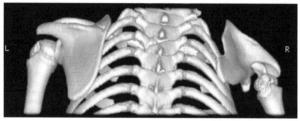

Figure 3.7. 3D-CT of patient with right OBPI. Acromion impingement on humeral head and abnormal migration of scapula and clavicle are evident in anterior view (top). Elevation and hypoplasia of scapula can be seen in posterior view (bottom). L indicates left, R indicates right.

modification of Mallet's classification system to index active shoulder movement[15]. In order to more precisely define functional disability, the angles of hand-to-mouth movement (trumpeter's sign) and forearm supination secondary to external rotation are recorded. The presence of a supinated forearm in the face of a medially rotated arm (see box on arm rotated medially with supination deformity) must be recognized and is defined in my application of the modified Mallet system. All clinical evaluations are videotaped and digitized.

The diagnosis of SHEAR deformity can be made clinically, but it is best defined with three-dimensional reconstruction of CT scans through the shoulder girdle. The method of Waters[8] is used on preoperative axial CT or Upright MRI images to grade GH deformity and subluxation. 3D-CT is used to determine severity of the underlying SHEAR deformity (see Ch. 4 for full description of methods for measuring and classifying SHEAR).

Positional *MRI*

The availability of positional (upright) MRI imaging of the glenohumeral joints allow a truer view of the joint when the arm is in the normal position of function. Traditional scanning, either CT or MRI, places patients into the recumbent position after which shoulder anatomy becomes subject to gravity in a non-functional position. The recumbent position creates false-negative impressions of the shoulder joint's dynamic anatomy and under-reports the presence of dislocations and subluxations of the humeral head.

As an example, the 15-year old patient shown was diagnosed on multiple occasions with a congruent shoulder joint by recumbent CT scan. This dissuaded his local physicians from operating on the joint

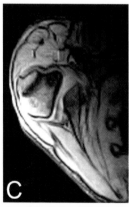

or the shoulder muscles and resulted in lack of abduction (A). However, positional scanning of the right shoulder joint (C) showed a complete dislocation of the humeral head while the patient was upright, allowing me to perform appropriate surgery to improve the active range of motion (B), even after many years of undiagnosed dislocation. The results should improve with time and earlier diagnosis in these situations should result in even better outcomes.

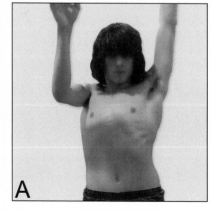

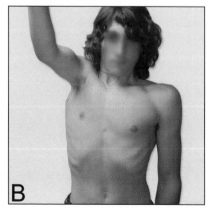

Treatment

Because of the rapid limb development taking place in neonatal brachial plexus patients, relatively minor functional limitations that result from brachial plexus injuries of the upper trunk may manifest themselves as serious deformities with lifelong disability. Ideally, early treatment may entail physical and occupational therapy, daily passive range of motion exercises, BTX-A injections and/or splinting to prevent the occurrence of biceps/triceps co-contraction[16, 17]. Often, however, deformations occur that require surgical intervention. Tightness in the axilla and pectoralis muscles must be treated early and aggressively for the best outcomes.

There are several opinions regarding the optimum treatment of residual functional limitation in OBPI. Some surgeons do not perform releases of muscle tightness in the setting of diagnosed underlying incongruent GH articulation because surgical releases and transfers are thought to promote anterior dislocation with external rotation-abduction contracture[18-20].

In my experience, neither anterior dislocations nor external rotation-abduction contractures have been noted in any of my patients who have undergone release and transfer treatments for muscle tightness. The noted complications are probably due to the presence of unrecognized SHEAR deformity and humeral head impingement by the tilted ACT.

Recumbent CT scanning has not been a consistently effective technique for the diagnosis of GH incongruity (see box on Upright MRI). In one experimental series that I analyzed, the majority of radiologists did not diagnose the presence of subluxation. The same may be true of recumbent MRI evaluation of subluxation and dislocation, although glenoid version is reliably diagnosed and measured.

The abduction deficit is effectively improved with soft tissue procedures, the most effective of which is the Quad surgery (Table 2.II). What has been more difficult to correct is the medial rotation due to the SHEAR deformity. The traditional approach has been the use of derotational humeral osteotomy to improve the position of the hand and forearm[18, 19, 21, 22]. Humeral osteotomy may provide a level of functional improvement (Table 3.I), but the procedure does not address the GH deformity or aim to correct shoulder dynamics. It simply places the arm in a more functional position and does not account for the presence of SHEAR deformity and its resultant motion-limiting impingement.

Table 3.I *Comparison of Humeral Osteotomy (1-7) to Triangle Tilt (present study)*

Author	Year	n	Age (range)	Location of rotation	Follow-up in years (range)	Improvement in abduction (Degree) Mallet	Improvement in external rotation (Degree) Mallet	Hand to Neck Pre Post	Hand to Mouth Pre Post	Average Mallet Pre Post	Total Mallet Pre Post
1. *Faysse*[26]	1972	51	8.5 (2.5-20)	30 superior and 21 inferior to deltoid insertion						1.8 / 2.8	
2. *Goddard*[27]	1984	10	7.7 (3.2-12.6)	superior to deltoid insertion	4.5 (2-8)	(9°) / None	(-69°) / 2 pts				
3. *Kirkos*[19]	1998	22	10.25 (4-17)	between subscapularis and pectoralis major insertions	(2-31)	(27°)	(66°) / 2			1.2 / 3	
4. *Al-Qattan*[18]	2002	15	6.5 (5-10)	inferior to deltoid insertion	3 (1-5)	(15°) / 4	1.8	2.2 / 4	2 / 3	2.6 / 3.7	
5. *Okcu*[28]	2003	20	8.1 (5-13)	distal border of the pectoralis major tendon	8	1	2	2 / 4	2 / 4	2.3 / 4	
6. *Akinci*[29]	2005	40	7.5 (2-14.8)	distal border of the pectoralis major tendon		(15.7°) / 1				2.1 / 4	
7. *Waters*[22]	2006	27	7.6 (2.3-17)	superior to deltoid insertion	3.7 (2-7.8)	0.5	1.2	2.6 / 3.7	2.7 / 4	2.7 / 3.6	13.3 / 18.2
8. **Nath**[30]	**2007**	**38**	**6.4 (2.2-10.3)**	**not applicable**	**1.3 (1.0-1.7)**	**0.2**	**1**	**2.4 / 3.6**	**1.8 / 3.8**	**2.8 / 3.7**	**13.6 / 18.6**

Additionally, by abandoning the humeral head in its abnormal position within the glenoid fossa, there is no opportunity for normalization of the joint's development. Serial scanning of the glenoid fossa before and after humeral osteotomy confirms persistence of glenoid deformity after this surgical procedure[22]. Humeral osteotomy either above or below the deltoid insertion does not address the GH derangement[13].

Another surgical procedure, the anterior GH capsule release, on its own, simply rotates the humerus within an abnormal glenoid without attempting to address the abnormal structure and angles of the scapula and glenoid fossa. There is a high risk of unsatisfactory external rotation deformity which is difficult to treat and may be functionally more limiting than the medial rotation contracture the procedure is designed to address. This is actually described by Pearl et al., the foremost proponents of the anterior capsule release[23]. However, the goal of GH centralization is valid and seems to result in improved glenoid anatomy following normalization of the humeral head within the fossa[23].

Posterior GH capsulorrhaphy tightens the posterior capsule surrounding the humeral head and repositions it anteriorly, but again, does not take into account the SHEAR deformity and its central influence in the pathophysiology of the medial rotation contracture. In my experience, on its own, posterior capsulorrhaphy has a high failure rate, as is predictable when taking the SHEAR into consideration.

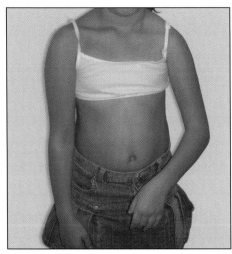

Figure 3.8. Seven-year old patient with severe left OBPI who previously underwent humeral derotational osteotomy at another institution. Recurrence of medial rotation is evident. At time of photograph, external rotation, supination and hand to back motions were impossible with left arm; patient also had difficulty with hand to head movements. Treatment with Triangle Tilt surgery was successful.

The presence of an unrecognized, high-grade SHEAR deformity can certainly lead to recurrence of the medial rotation deformity after humeral osteotomy (Figure 3.8) and is related to ongoing impingement of the distal ACT against the humeral head. The curious fact that in several published clinical series of derotational humeral osteotomy, the exis-

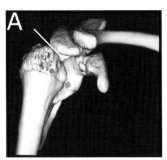
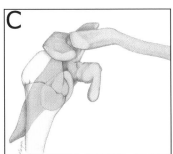
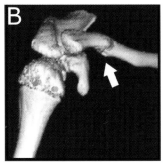
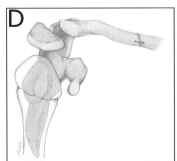

Figure 3.9. 3D-CT (left) and artist's rendering (right) of AC interface before (top) and after (bottom) Triangle Tilt surgery. In A, the thin white line shows the impingement between the acromion process and the humeral head due to the abnormally elevated scapula. During Triangle Tilt, this is corrected by detaching the distal acromion from the scapular spine. Osteotomy of the clavicle (white arrow, B) allows it to unwind back to a neutral position. As a result, the humeral head has been relocated into the glenoid fossa, with a neutral position. The 3D-CT images show the correction of both the posterior subluxation of the humeral head and the internal rotation of the humeral head (blue and green dots) within the glenoid fossa (red dot) that is achieved by this procedure. In B, the glenoid fossa cannot be seen, as GHJ congruency has been restored (represented by overlap of the green and red dots). This should allow more normal development of the shoulder joint.

tence of similar obvious recurrences is not mentioned, leads to concern about the application of functional grading systems.

In my hands, successful restoration of position and function in failed humeral osteotomy patients has followed from surgically addressing the SHEAR deformity. It may be inferred that the SHEAR correction (the Triangle Tilt surgery, see below) is a superior operation because it addresses the root cause of the medial rotation. Further, this result indicates that the SHEAR deformity is indeed the underlying pathophysiology behind the fixed medial rotation deformity.

Triangle Tilt Surgery

The summary evaluation of the material presented above is that a novel approach is required to take into account the presence of the SHEAR deformity in most, if not all, cases of medial rotation contracture. Conceptually, a bony surgical procedure would detach the distal ACT-humeral head complex from the abnormally positioned scapula; subsequent reversal of the anterior tilt of the ACT then would allow a natural rotation of the humeral head back into a more neutral position within the glenoid fossa.

In practice, this concept requires osteotomies of the clavicle and neck of the acromion. This releases the distal triangle and allows it to tilt back to its neutral position, in essence a leveling movement of the triangle (Figure 3.9). The surgical procedure is accordingly named the "Triangle Tilt."

The release and tilting of the acromio-clavicular plane back to neutral appears to relieve the impingement of the ACT on the humeral head and allows the head to be repositioned passively into a neutral position within the glenoid fossa (Figure 3.9). This should improve the favorable chances of maintained long-term function.

The importance of recognizing and diagnosing the presence of a SHEAR deformity in MRC patients cannot be emphasized enough. If SHEAR is present, it must be accounted for in both the surgical and treatment plans.

Surgical Procedure

The Triangle Tilt surgery consists of:

(1) osteotomy of the clavicle at the junction of the middle and distal thirds

(2) osteotomy of the acromion process at its junction with the spine of the scapula

(3) ostectomy of the superomedial angle of the scapula to reduce scapular winging

(4) splinting of the extremity in adduction, external rotation and forearm supination

Minor elements of the procedure include bone grafting of the acromion process and clavicular osteotomy sites and semi-rigid fixation of the clavicular osteotomy segments to prevent nonunion. Posterior GH capsulorrhaphy and/or anterior GH capsule release is performed in cases of shoulder instability diagnosed by preoperative, positional MRI

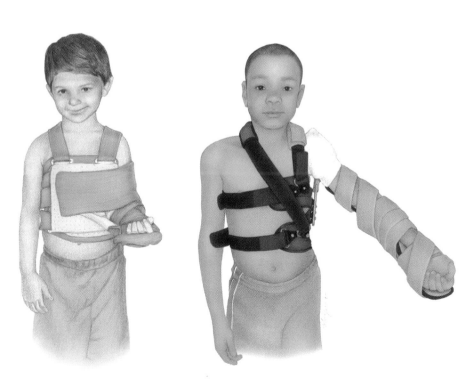

Figure 3.10. Patients are placed into either a "gunslinger" splint (pictured, left) or a SARO brace (Becker Orthopedic; pictured, right) after Triangle Tilt surgery. The gunslinger splint maintains the arm in full adduction, the humerus in a neutral and externally rotated position and the forearm in supination during healing. The SARO brace maintains the arm in partial adduction, the elbow in extension and the forearm in supination. To minimize loss of medial rotation, I do not splint the arm in full external (lateral) rotation. The type of splint used depends on the individual patient's problem.

3 | *Bone Deformities & Their Management*

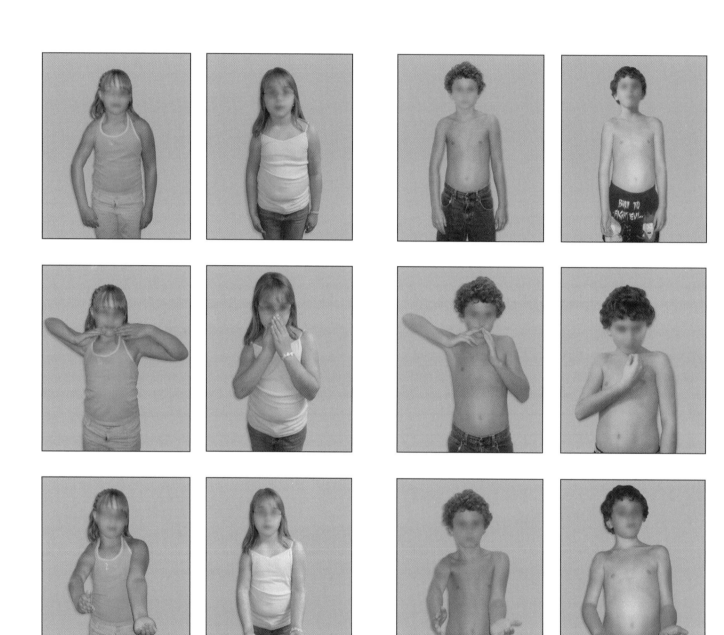

Figure 3.11. Triangle Tilt improves resting position, hand to mouth motions and supination. A 9-year old girl having had previous primary nerve grafting of the brachial plexus as an infant and contracture release surgery (Mod Quad) nevertheless shows the characteristic movement patterns of SHEAR deformity (left pictures). Correction by Triangle Tilt surgery was successful (right pictures).

Figure 3.12. Improvements seen after Triangle Tilt. A 12-year old boy who has had no previous surgery shows the characteristic movement patterns of SHEAR deformity (left pictures). Correction by Triangle Tilt surgery (right pictures) was successful. Note the similarities in deformity and Triangle Tilt results between this patient and that shown in Figure 3.11, who underwent two surgeries, including nerve grafting, prior to Triangle Tilt.

imaging in conjunction with the physical examination. Postoperative splinting (Figure 3.10) is maintained for 6 weeks; subsequently, the splint is worn only at night for an additional 6-12 months.

Evidence of Triangle Tilt Surgery Effectiveness

Immediately after osteotomy of the clavicle, unwinding of the distal and proximal clavicle segments occurs, reflecting the abnormal twist of the clavicle that takes place secondary to scapular migration. Moreover, following osteotomy of the acromion process, the distal segment immediately moves both inferiorly and posteriorly as the distal acromial head and the proximal acromial neck separate. The rapid clavicular and acromial movements after osteotomy are evidence of the highly abnormal bony framework surrounding the injured shoulder and the significant intraosseous torque that is released upon separating the distal ACT from the abnormally medial structures. As part of the GHJ, the humeral head is related to the lateral structures and, therefore, becomes normalized along with the distal ACT. This produces a new environment that is free of abnormal deforming torque within the bony skeleton of the shoulder.

The Triangle Tilt procedure was designed to eliminate the impingement on the humeral head that results from the SHEAR deformity and to improve the position of the humeral head in the glenoid. It is known that progressive glenohumeral dysplasia occurs in children with OBPI[8, 12]. The progressive dysplasia observed in the glenoid is comparable to that observed in the acetabulum in development of dysplasia of the hip[12]. In the hip joint, osseous procedures that tilt the acetabulum have been used to correct poor positioning of the femur[24] with early intervention providing better results[25]. Analogously, surgical adjustment of the plane of the distal spino-clavicular triangle, as performed in the Triangle Tilt procedure, is a rational approach to address the glenohumeral deformity of OBPI. Improved glenohumeral anatomy should lead to long-term improvement of shoulder function.

Recently, I reviewed 40 of my OBPI patients with persistent medial rotation deformity. The patients were selected consecutively. None of the patients had had previous bony surgery. Ten had undergone primary nerve surgery in infancy. Posterior glenohumeral capsulorrhaphy surgery was attempted on ten (all ten failed). All 40 patients had previously undergone the Mod Quad procedure that improved

abduction by at least 90° (mean 160°, maximum 180°). However, the resting medial rotation posture persisted and was not responsive to therapy and splinting.

The mean Mallet score of these patients improved from 13.6 points (range: 9 to 19) preoperatively to 18.6 points (range: 14 to 22) ($p<0.001$) at an average of 15 months after Triangle Tilt surgery (Table 3.I). Hand to mouth movements occurred in an improved functional plane: mean trumpet sign angle significantly decreased (preoperatively: mean 110°, range 60° to 160°; postoperatively: mean 36°, range 0° to 100°; $p<0.001$). Supination of the forearm (actually a function of improved shoulder external rotation) increased (preoperatively: mean -12°, range -80° to 50°; postoperatively: mean 36°, range -45° to 90°; $p<0.001$). The mean active global range of shoulder movement was not significantly affected (postoperative mean 165°, range 90° to 180°).

As shown (Figures 3.11-3.12), Triangle Tilt patients demonstrated noticeable improvement in hand to mouth movements and supination. Arm posture in the resting position also significantly improved. The preoperative medial rotation caused the arm to flare laterally in the resting position; in this posture, the elbow was held in flexion. The surgical leveling of the ACT moved the glenohumeral axis toward neutral and significantly improved clinical arm position and movement. Correction of the flaring of the arm contributed to the visible improvement. In this way, the Triangle Tilt serves a similar function to derotational humeral osteotomy but has the added benefit of being more physiological and results in normalized glenohumeral anatomy. Moreover, because it directly addresses the scapular deformity that is the pathophysiological basis for the medial rotation contracture, it is superior to both anterior capsule release and humeral osteotomy.

Postoperative CT images available for two patients in this series showed improvement in GH congruency (Figure 3.13). In these cases, the head of the humerus was relocated within the glenoid fossa to a more natural position, indicating correction of the medial rotation deformity. The posterior GH capsulorrhaphy resolves the posterior laxity caused by humeral head displacement.

In summary, the improvement in overall Mallet score, an average of 4.9, seen after Triangle Tilt surgery is superior to the published results of humeral osteotomy and anterior capsule release (Table 3.I)[23]. This is largely due to improved hand to mouth motion (decreased trumpeter's sign). Significant improvement is also seen in hand to neck and hand to spine movements ($p<0.001$). These are the move-

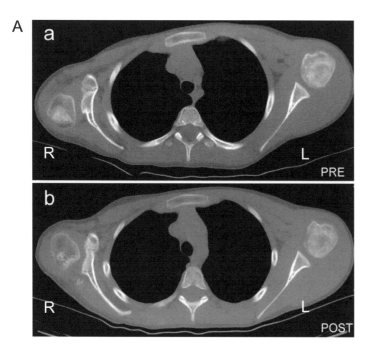

A

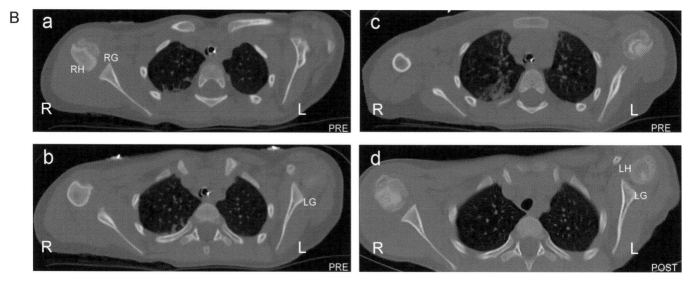

B

Figure 3.13. Triangle Tilt restores glenohumeral congruency.
A. (a) Axial CT images of nine-year old patient with severe glenohumeral deformity and posterior humeral subluxation of the right arm; (b) axial CT of the same patient taken after Triangle Tilt surgery demonstrates the noticeable improvement in glenohumeral congruency achieved by this procedure. B. Axial CT scans of five-year old patient with left OBPI showing glenohumeral deformity and inferior humeral subluxation of the affected shoulder. (a) Congruent right glenohumeral joint; (b-c) CT images obtained from two different axial planes show an incongruent left glenohumeral joint with glenoid and humeral head deformities. Due to inferior humeral subluxation, the affected humeral head (c) and glenoid (b) do not appear on the same plane. (d) After Triangle Tilt surgery, restoration of left glenohumeral congruency can be seen, right and left glenohumeral joints appear in the same axial plane. R indicates right, L indicates left, H indicates humeral head, G indicates glenoid.

ments addressed by humeral osteotomy and anterior capsule release. The sensitivity of Mallet functional scoring is not sufficient to discriminate subtle differences in all patients, thus additional measurements of hand to mouth and supination angles were made. These both showed significant improvement following Triangle Tilt surgery. It is expected that by directly addressing the underlying SHEAR deformity in these patients, improvements will be better maintained than improvements seen due to surgeries which do not address the SHEAR. In addition, minimal progression of GHJ deformity is expected.

Literature Cited

1. Birch R, Bonney G, Wynn Parry CB. Birth lesions of the brachial plexus. In: Birch R, Bonney G, Wynn Parry CB, eds. *Surgical disorders of the peripheral nerves.* New York, NY: Churchill Livingstone; 1998:209-233.

2. Bubenik GA, Bubenik AB, Stevens ED, Binnington AG. The effect of neurogenic stimulation on the development and growth of bony tissues. *J Exp Zool.* Feb 1 1982;219(2):205-216.

3. Edoff K, Hellman J, Persliden J, Hildebrand C. The developmental skeletal growth in the rat foot is reduced after denervation. *Anat Embryol (Berl).* Jun 1997;195(6):531-538.

4. Garcia-Castellano JM, Diaz-Herrera P, Morcuende JA. Is bone a target-tissue for the nervous system? New advances on the understanding of their interactions. *Iowa Orthop J.* 2000;20:49-58.

5. Hukkanen M, Konttinen YT, Santavirta S, et al. Rapid proliferation of calcitonin gene-related peptide-immunoreactive nerves during healing of rat tibial fracture suggests neural involvement in bone growth and remodelling. *Neuroscience.* Jun 1993;54(4):969-979.

6. Moukoko D, Ezaki M, Wilkes D, Carter P. Posterior shoulder dislocation in infants with neonatal brachial plexus palsy. *J Bone Joint Surg Am.* Apr 2004;86-A(4):787-793.

7. van der Sluijs JA, van Ouwerkerk WJ, de Gast A, Wuisman P, Nollet F, Manoliu RA. Retroversion of the humeral head in children with an obstetric brachial plexus lesion. *J Bone Joint Surg Br.* May 2002;84(4):583-587.

8. Waters PM, Smith GR, Jaramillo D. Glenohumeral deformity secondary to brachial plexus birth palsy. *J Bone Joint Surg Am.* May 1998;80(5):668-677.

9. Gudinchet F, Maeder P, Oberson JC, Schnyder P. Magnetic resonance imaging of the shoulder in children with brachial pLexus birth palsy. *Pediatr Radiol.* Nov 1995;25 Suppl 1:S125-128.

10. Hernandez RJ, Dias L. CT evaluation of the shoulder in children with Erb's palsy. *Pediatr Radiol.* 1988;18(4):333-336.

11. Hoeksma AF, Ter Steeg AM, Dijkstra P, Nelissen RG, Beelen A, de Jong BA. Shoulder contracture and osseous deformity in obstetrical brachial plexus injuries. *J Bone Joint Surg Am.* Feb 2003;85-A(2):316-322.

12. Pearl ML, Edgerton BW. Glenoid deformity secondary to brachial plexus birth palsy. *J Bone Joint Surg Am.* May 1998;80(5):659-667.

13. Kambhampati SB, Birch R, Cobiella C, Chen L. Posterior subluxation and dislocation of the shoulder in obstetric brachial plexus palsy. *J Bone Joint Surg Br.* Feb 2006;88(2):213-219.

14. Birch R. Medial rotation contracture and posterior dislocation of the shoulder. In: Gilbert A, ed. *Brachial plexus injuries.* First ed. London: Martin Dunitz, Ltd.; 2001:249-259.

15. Mallet J. [Obstetrical paralysis of the brachial plexus. II. Therapeutics. Treatment of sequelae. e. Results of different therapeutic techniques and therapeutic indications]. *Rev Chir Orthop Reparatrice Appar Mot.* 1972;58:Suppl 1:192-196.

16. Rollnik JD, Hierner R, Schubert M, et al. Botulinum toxin treatment of cocontractions after birth-related brachial plexus lesions. *Neurology.* Jul 12 2000;55(1):112-114.

17. Waters PM. Update on management of pediatric brachial plexus palsy. *J Pediatr Orthop B.* Jul 2005;14(4):233-244.

18. Al-Qattan MM. Rotation osteotomy of the humerus for Erb's palsy in children with humeral head deformity. *J Hand Surg [Am].* May 2002;27(3):479-483.

19. Kirkos JM, Papadopoulos IA. Late treatment of brachial plexus palsy secondary to birth injuries: rotational osteotomy of the proximal part of the humerus. *J Bone Joint Surg Am.* Oct 1998;80(10):1477-1483.

20. Zancolli EA. Classification and management of the shoulder in birth palsy. *Orthop Clin North Am.* Apr 1981;12(2):433-457.

21. Egloff DV, Raffoul W, Bonnard C, Stalder J. Palliative surgical procedures to restore shoulder function in obstetric brachial palsy. Critical analysis of Narakas' series. *Hand Clin.* Nov 1995;11(4):597-606.

22. Waters PM, Bae DS. The effect of derotational humeral osteotomy on global shoulder function in brachial plexus birth palsy. *J Bone Joint Surg Am.* May 2006;88(5):1035-1042.

23. Pearl ML, Edgerton BW, Kazimiroff PA, Burchette RJ, Wong K. Arthroscopic release and latissimus dorsi transfer for shoulder internal rotation contractures and glenohumeral deformity secondary to brachial plexus birth palsy. *J Bone Joint Surg Am.* Mar 2006;88(3):564-574.

24. Hartofilakidis G, Stamos K, Karachalios T, Ioannidis TT, Zacharakis N. Congenital hip disease in adults. Classification of acetabular deficiencies and operative treatment with acetabuloplasty combined with total hip arthroplasty. *J Bone Joint Surg Am.* May 1996;78(5):683-692.

25. Lalonde FD, Frick SL, Wenger DR. Surgical correction of residual hip dysplasia in two pediatric age-groups. *J Bone Joint Surg Am.* Jul 2002;84-A(7):1148-1156.

26. Faysse R. [Obstetrical paralysis of the bronchial plexus. II. Therapeutics. Treatment of sequelae. d. Humeral derotation osteotomy in the sequelae]. *Rev Chir Orthop Reparatrice Appar Mot.* 1972;58:Suppl 1:187-192.

27. Goddard NJ, Fixsen JA. Rotation osteotomy of the humerus for birth injuries of the brachial plexus. *J Bone Joint Surg Br.* Mar 1984;66(2):257-259.

28. Okcu G, Kapubağli A. [Lateral humeral rotation osteotomy for the treatment of obstetrical palsy of the brachial plexus]. [*Clinical Research. Turkey*]. 2003;14(3):146-152.

29. Akinci M, Ay S, Kamiloglu S, Ercetin O. [External rotation osteotomy of the humerus for the treatment of shoulder problems secondary to obstetric brachial plexus palsy]. *Acta Orthop Traumatol Turc.* 2005;39(4):328-333.

30. Data submitted for publication. Also refer to Nath RK, Melcher SE, Paizi M. Surgical correction of unsuccessful derotational humeral osteotomy in obstetric brachial plexus palsy: Evidence of the significance of scapular deformity in the pathophysiology of the medial rotation contracture. *J Brachial Plex Peripher Nerve Inj.* 2006;1:9.

Chapter 4   Measurement & Classification of SHEAR Deformity

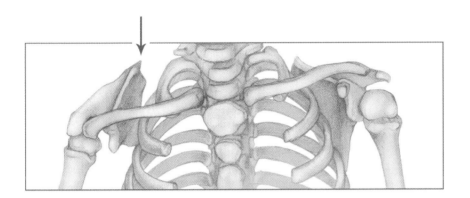

Introduction

Muscles that stabilize the shoulder girdle are supplied by the fifth cervical root. Because it is the most common brachial plexus nerve root affected in obstetric injuries, shoulder deformities are the most common of the OBPI sequelae. The pathophysiology of this deformity has been described in previous chapters. Previous radiologic studies of scapular deformities have been reported but they generally focused on the glenoid fossa and adjacent structures[1-4]. During my examinations of thousands of OBPI patients, I observed that a significant percentage developed several common changes to the shape, size and position of the shoulder girdle that had not been previously described in the literature. Based on these observations, I initiated a study that focused on the body, spine and acromion process of the scapula to accurately characterize this deformity[5].

Patients with SHEAR deformity have unilateral scapular elevation as a result of upward migration of the scapula. The position of the affected scapula does not have the characteristics of Sprengel's deformity, which is a congenital origin of scapular elevation. The hypoplasia of the scapula results from the brachial plexus injury and the apparent elevation is the result of rotation about an axis perpendicular to the scapular plane.

Measurement and Grading of SHEAR

Bilateral axial CT images and three dimensional reconstructions of data from tomograms (3D-CT) are used in the evaluation process. Injured shoulder girdles are examined on anterior and posterior trunk views as well as superior trunk outlet, scapular posterior and medial views. The contralateral scapula is always assessed for comparison. The measurement parameters used to assess shoulder deformity are summarized in Table 4.I and demonstrated in Figure 4.1.

It is repeatedly observed that the area of scapula visible above the clavicle is increased in OBPI patients with shoulder deformity. Based on this observation, the correlation of each measurement parameter (Table 4.I) with the area of the scapula visible above the clavicle was evaluated to characterize the scapular deformity.

A grading scale to assess scapular deformity in brachial plexus palsy was devised by calculating the percentages of different parts of the scapula visible above the clavicle on 3D-CTs of my patients. The stages of deformity are detailed in Table 4.II. The SHEAR grades range from 0-4, the most severe cases of SHEAR receiving a score of 4. Representative cases for each grade are illustrated in Figure 4.2.

Mechanism of SHEAR

Loss of innervation to target muscles, resulting from birth injury, causes the muscles to become weak. Due to the relationship between mechanical loading of bones and bone formation, the affected scapula is not only malpositioned, it is also hypoplastic. Weakened scapular stabilizer muscles are not capable of applying substantial forces to the scapula, leading to a decreased rate of bone growth[1, 2]. This is supported by measurements of total area of the scapula; the

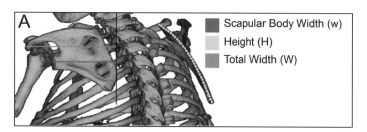

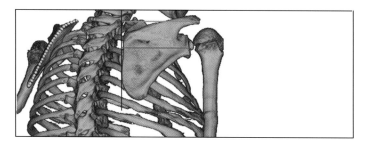

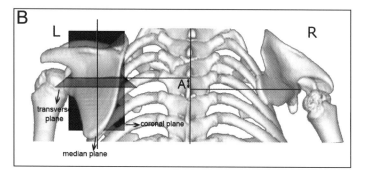

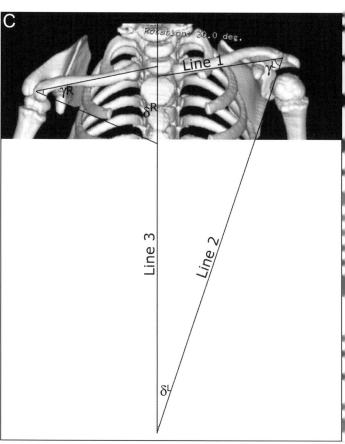

Figure 4.1. SHEAR Measurements. A. Scapular height and width measurements on scapular view of 3D-CT. Measurements indicated on left scapula with SHEAR deformity (top) and normal right shoulder (bottom). B. Vertical displacement and anatomical planes on posterior trunk view. C. Anterior trunk view used to measure inferior scapular angle (δ) and superior scapular angle (γ). Notice increase in δ and decrease in γ due to SHEAR. L indicates left; R indicates right.

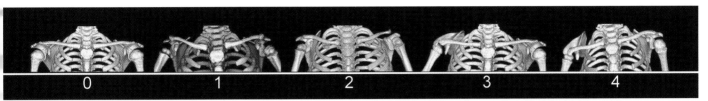

Figure 4.2. 3D-CT of representative cases of each grade of SHEAR deformity as detailed in Table 4.II.

total area of the hypoplastic scapula averages 14% less than the contralateral scapula and correlates with the severity of the deformity (r=-0.57).

While the overall growth (height and width) of the body of the scapula is impaired after OBPI, the acromion follows a normal growth rate. In some cases, the deformity is more severe and the acromion grows at an increased aberrant rate that causes it to impinge upon the humeral head.

In cases of congenital scapular elevation (Sprengel's deformity), the severity of the deformity correlates with the level of the shoulder joint[6]. However, vertical displacement measurements in OBPI patients indicate that the apparent elevation of the scapula is the result of rotational displacement. In most cases, the rotation about a vertical axis is internal and the rotation about the axis of the scapular spine is anterior, causing a narrowing of the scapuloclavicular space on the superior trunk outlet view.

Table 4.I *Definitions of SHEAR Measurements*[*]

Hypoplasia	
Height of scapula (H)	Scapular medial view, length of medial border between the superior angle and the inferior angle.
Total width (W)	Measured from the lateral end of the acromion to the most medial part of the scapula (Figure 4.1A).
Width of the body of the scapula (w)	Measured as the distance from the glenoid to the most medial part of the scapula (Figure 4.1A).
Total area of the scapula	Calculated on scapular posterior view (Figure 4.1A).
Downward/Upward Rotation of scapula (about the median plane)	Defined by the angle between the extension of the line connecting the mid glenoid to the base of the spine of the scapula and the vertebral axis line.
Superior scapular angle (γ)	Angle defined between lines 1[A] and 2[A].
Inferior scapular angle (δ)	Angle between lines 2 and 3[A] (Figure 4.1C).
Vertical displacement	Percentage of the difference between the levels of the two glenoids (A) divided by the height of the contralateral scapula (H). Positive sign denotes superior displacement and negative sign inferior displacement (Figure 4.1B) (measured on the trunk posterior view). Lines drawn from center of glenoid cavity perpendicularly to the vertebral axis line.
Internal/external rotation (about the coronal plane)	Defined by the angle between scapular line[B] and the vertebral axis (spinoscapular angle).
Anterior/Posterior rotation (about the transverse plane)	Assessed on the superior outlet view by measuring the angle of convergence of the longitudinal lines of the shaft of the clavicle and the line connecting the superomedial angle of the scapula to the acromio-clavicular joint.
Area of the scapula visible on the anterior view above the clavicle (with reference to the contralateral side)	Measured on the trunk anterior view. For distance and area measurements, graphic software (Universal Desktop Ruler, AVPSoft.com) is used.
Glenoscapular angle (glenoid version)	Measured according to Friedman et al [13] as the angle between the scapular line[B] and the line connecting the base of the anterior labrum and posterior labrum. By definition 90° is subtracted from the posteromedial quadrant angle to define the glenoscapular angle.
Percentage of subluxation	Percentage of the greatest diameter of the humeral head and the distance of the scapular line to the anterior portion of the head[4].

Table Legend
*Both the affected and contralateral sides are assessed and the values discussed take into account comparison between sides unless specifically indicated. Descriptive statistics are calculated for each variable, including mean, standard deviation and range. Comparisons of means for continuous variables are performed by the Pearson product correlation coefficients and the paired Student's t-test with Microsoft Excel 2003 software (Microsoft, Redmond, WA). P values are two-tailed, and p values of <0.05 are considered to be significant.
A: Two angles are calculated between three lines forming a triangle: Line 1 is drawn between the sterno-clavicular joint and the center of the acromio-clavicular joint and line 2 between the center of the acromio-clavicular joint and the inferior angle of the scapula, Line 3 is the vertebral axis line.
B: scapular line connects the medial margin of the scapula to the middle of the glenoid fossa.

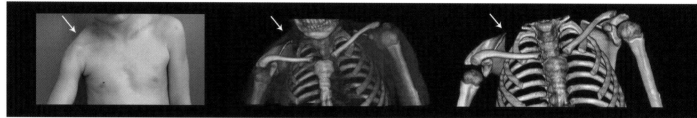

Figure 4.3. Visible effects of SHEAR deformity include sloping of involved shoulder.

As the scapula rotates, the position of the acromio-clavicular joint also changes. This contributes to impingement upon the humeral head by the distal acromion and clavicle, resulting in the MRC described above. The clinical implications of the MRC have been described by Birch in detail[7], and the discovery of the SHEAR deformity allows a rational treatment plan (such as the Triangle Tilt surgery) to be developed. The elevation and forward rotation of the scapula causes a sloping of the region between the shoulder and the neck (Figure 4.3)

Conclusions

During the development of scapular dysplasia, both rotational deformity (angle of the spine of the scapula) and decreased height to width ratio contribute to decreased superior scapular angle (γ) and increased inferior scapular angle (δ) (Figure 4.1C); both also strongly correlate with area of scapula visible above clavicle (r=-0.75 and r=0.83) and degree of subluxation (r=0.63 and r=-0.63).

My findings that SHEAR score, based on the percentage of scapula visible over the clavicle, strongly correlates with rotation and hypoplasia of the scapula and humeral subluxation, provides a convenient diagnostic tool. With the

pathophysiology established, anatomical correction of the deformity was considered and planned, with documented improvement in functional parameters.

Progressive glenoid deformity, reflected by altered glenoid version measurements, is a well-known tertiary effect of OBPI and has been discussed previously at length[8,9]. Global abduction has been correlated with glenoid version[4]. Other than global abduction, the literature does not indicate a significant correlation between Mallet functional parameters, and either radiographic parameters or age[4,9]. This is likely because active shoulder function is dependent upon the glenohumeral relationship, the integrity of the shoulder capsule, the strength and physical properties of the muscles and the nervous system.

It is clear that the SHEAR deformity is the most important cause of MRC and should, therefore, be the pathophysiologic basis for treatment of the problem. The Triangle Tilt surgery (see Chs. 3 and 5) offers a direct solution to the SHEAR deformity and addresses the subluxation that accompanies SHEAR. Previous research has shown that soft tissue surgical procedures, such as anterior capsule release (ACR), positively influence the development of the glenoid fossa, whereas humeral osteotomy does not[10,11]. Both these reconstructive methods fail to address the underlying pathophys-

Table 4.II *SHEAR Grading Criteria*

	0	1	2	3	4
Percent of scapula visible above clavicle	< 2.0	2.0 – 3.6	3.6-20	20-42	42-55
Percent of superior border visible above clavicle	<20	20-45	45-58	58-68	68-71
Percent of medial border above clavicle	<6.5	6.5-16.5	16.5-28	28-50.5	50.5-65

iology and have two unacceptable side effects: (1) excessive external rotation posture with the ACR and (2) persistent abduction loss and glenoid deformity with humeral osteotomy. My experience with the Triangle Tilt surgery shows improvement in Mallet grading superior to both ACR and humeral osteotomy, while allowing replacement of the humeral head within the glenoid fossa. The large majority of Triangle Tilt surgeries are done in patients who have previously benefited from the Mod Quad surgery and therefore have the best reported outcomes in abduction and external rotation along with the additional resolution of shoulder subluxation.

In summary, residual neurological deficit in obstetric brachial plexus patients leads to muscular imbalances about the shoulder which influence the growth of the supplied osteocartilagenous elements. Scapular deformities common to this population may be diagnosed and classified using the SHEAR grading criteria presented in Table 4.II, enabling objective evaluation of the bony deformity and its severity as guide for treatment[5,12].

Literature Cited

1.   Kattan K, Spitz HB. Roentgen findings in obstetrical injuries to the brachial plexus. *Radiology.* 1968;91:462-467.

2.   Pollock AN, Reed MH. Shoulder deformities from obstetrical brachial plexus paralysis. *Skeletal Radiol.* 1989;18(4):295-297.

3.   Terzis JK, Vekris MD, Okajima S, Soucacos PN. Shoulder deformities in obstetric brachial plexus paralysis: a computed tomography study. *J Pediatr Orthop.* Mar-Apr 2003;23(2):254-260.

4.   Waters PM, Smith GR, Jaramillo D. Glenohumeral deformity secondary to brachial plexus birth palsy. *J Bone Joint Surg Am.* May 1998;80(5):668-677.

5.   Nath RK, Paizi M. Scapular deformity in obstetric brachial plexus palsy: a new finding. *Surg Radiol Anat.* 2007;in press. DOI: 10.1007/s00276-006-0173-1.

6.   Cho TJ, Choi IH, Chung CY, Hwang JK. The Sprengel deformity. Morphometric analysis using 3D-CT and its clinical relevance. *J Bone Joint Surg Br.* Jul 2000;82(5):711-718.

7.   Birch R. Medial rotation contracture and posterior dislocation of the shoulder. In: Gilbert A, ed. *Brachial plexus injuries.* First ed. London: Martin Dunitz, Ltd.; 2001:249-259.

8.   Al-Qattan MM. Classification of secondary shoulder deformities in obstetric brachial plexus palsy. *J Hand Surg [Br].* Oct 2003;28(5):483-486.

9.   van der Sluijs JA, van der Meij M, Verbeke J, Manoliu RA, Wuisman PI. Measuring secondary deformities of the shoulder in children with obstetric brachial plexus lesion: reliability of three methods. *J Pediatr Orthop B.* May 2003;12(3):211-214.

10.   Pearl ML, Edgerton BW, Kazimiroff PA, Burchette RJ, Wong K. Arthroscopic release and latissimus dorsi transfer for shoulder internal rotation contractures and glenohumeral deformity secondary to brachial plexus birth palsy. *J Bone Joint Surg Am.* Mar 2006;88(3):564-574.

11.   Waters PM, Bae DS. The effect of derotational humeral osteotomy on global shoulder function in brachial plexus birth palsy. *J Bone Joint Surg Am.* May 2006;88(5):1035-1042.

12.   Hartofilakidis G, Stamos K, Karachalios T, Ioannidis TT, Zacharakis N. Congenital hip disease in adults. Classification of acetabular deficiencies and operative treatment with acetabuloplasty combined with total hip arthroplasty. *J Bone Joint Surg Am.* May 1996;78(5):683-692.

13.   Friedman RJ, Hawthorne KB, Genez BM. The use of computerized tomography in the measurement of glenoid version. *J Bone Joint Surg Am.* Aug 1992;74(7):1032-1037.

Chapter 5 15 QUESTIONS for OBPI
Patient Evaluation

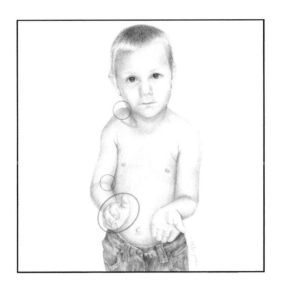

Introduction

There are over 500,000 combinations of treatable clinical presentations possible with Erb's palsy. This has confounded clinical evaluations of OBPI patients and hindered the development of standard treatment protocols. In an effort to address this issue, I have developed the "15 questions" system that serves as the basis for clinical decision making in my practice.

This concept is based on the fifteen most common and treatable deformities that occur with OBPI. Each of the questions describes an abnormality that inhibits function. Each of the fifteen deformities has a clear surgical and therapeutic solution. The most important clinical complications are identified by this system, in my experience.

15 QUESTIONS for OBPI Patient Evaluation

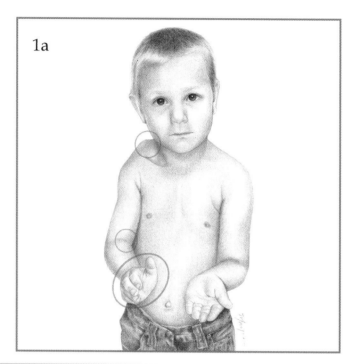

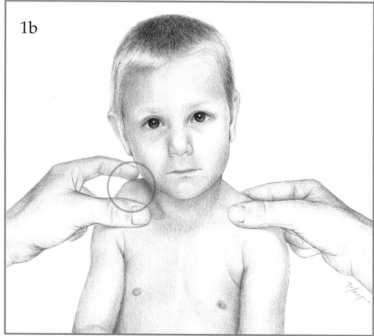

Question 1: Is the scapula elevated? Diagnosis is made by viewing the scapula rising on attempted supination (Figure 5.1a) as well as noting the difficulty in supination. Palpation of the clavicle with the thumb and the spine of the scapula with the index finger shows the upward tilt of the triangle between the clavicle and the acromion (tip of the scapula) on the child's right side (Figure 5.1b) compared with the uninjured left side. Circles mark areas of interest.

Treatment: Question 1

Scapular elevation is a critical element in the pathophysiology of the medial rotation contracture. This causes impingement of the acromion process and the distal clavicle on the humeral head, resulting in the abnormalities of movement characteristic of the deformity (flared elbow, lack of obvious supination, loss of external rotation at the shoulder, shortening of the arm, and often biceps contracture and dislocated radial head).

The scapular elevation is probably related to rhomboid weakness and this moves the humeral head and shaft into their abnormal positions by connections from the ligaments of the acromio-clavicular joint to the glenohumeral joint. Since there is no good way to reposition the scapula into its more natural medial position, treatment is aimed at separating the humeral head from the abnormal scapula.

Treatment requires the **Triangle Tilt** surgery (see Ch. 3.).

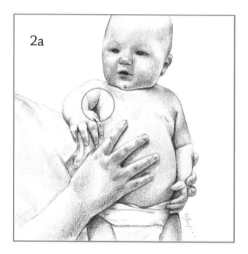

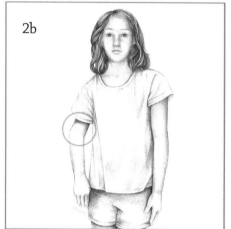

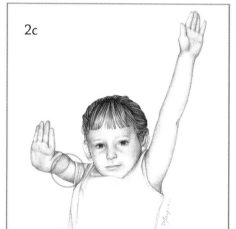

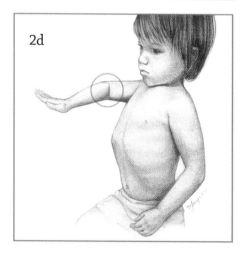

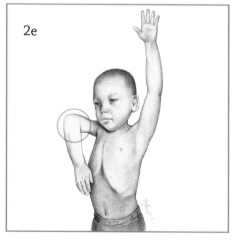

Question 2: Is the arm medially rotated? Diagnosis is made by viewing the elbow crease at rest (Figure 5.2a and 5.2b). Note that the elbow crease on the child's injured right side is not visible to the same extent as the uninjured side. The elbow crease often points directly sideways toward the chest (Figure 5.2c and 5.2d) compared with the uninjured left side. When a weak triceps is present, the elbow crease may point backward (Figure 5.2e). Circles mark areas of interest.

Treatment: Question 2

Medial rotation of the arm is a common feature of children with brachial plexus injury. The cause is the SHEAR deformity (see Ch. 4) of scapular elevation and rotation. Traditional treatment has been aimed at rotating the humerus away from the midline (Derotational Humeral Osteotomy) but this has a failure rate and also does not address the shoulder joint deformity. Another approach, the anterior capsule release (ACR) results in unacceptable loss of medial rotation. Both humeral osteotomy and ACR do not address the SHEAR deformity as the underlying cause of the problem.

Note that this is a failure of horizontal movement of the shoulder joint and is caused by bony deformities. Therefore, treatment is through bony surgery.

Treatment requires the **Triangle Tilt** surgery (see Ch. 3).

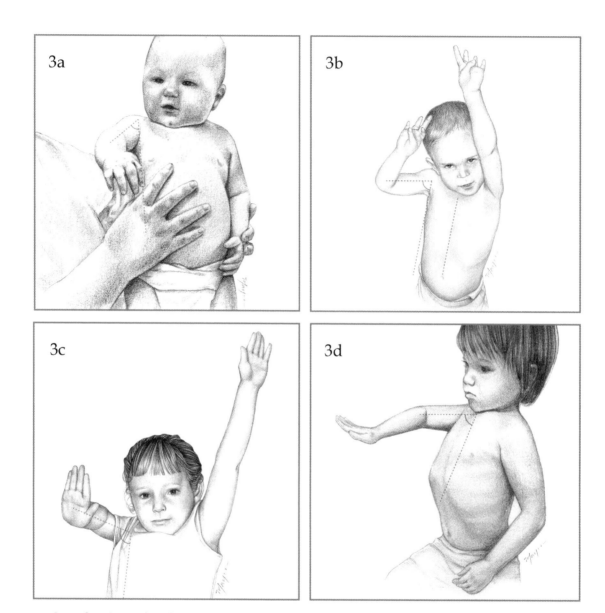

Question 3: Is the shoulder active range of motion less than 120 degrees? Diagnosis is made by viewing the angle between the trunk axis and the axis of the injured arm (Figure 5.3a, 5.3b, 5.3c and 5.3d). Comparison with the opposite side is useful as well. In Figure 5.3a, 5.3c, and 5.3d, abnormal truncal flexion is seen and should be accounted for in making measurements.

Treatment: Question 3

The bony SHEAR deformity causes loss of horizontal movements of the shoulder joint, resulting in external rotation and supination deficits. Loss of the vertical component of shoulder mobility is due to contractures of the muscles of the axilla and chest (see Ch. 2.)

Difficulty in abduction and flexion of the shoulder is best treated in my experience by surgical contracture releases and muscle transfers, which are soft tissue procedures. When there is loss of *active* overhead movement that is significant, at around 120 degrees, surgery is indicated.

Treatment requires the **Modified Quad** surgery (see Ch. 2).

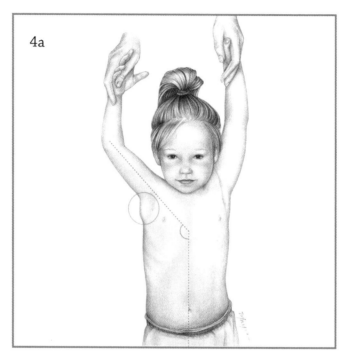

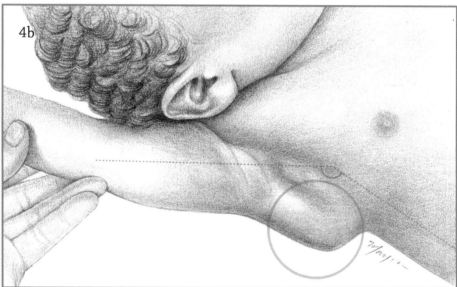

Question 4: Is the passive range of motion of the shoulder less than 150 degrees?
Diagnosis is made by viewing the angle between the trunk axis and the axis of the injured arm (Figure 5.4a and 5.4b). Comparison with the opposite side is useful as well. In Figure 5.4a and 5.4b, lateral winging of the scapula is noted on passive movement of the arm into abduction. Circles mark areas of interest.

Treatment: Question 4

The bony SHEAR deformity causes loss of horizontal movements of the shoulder joint, resulting in external rotation and supination deficits. Loss of the vertical component of shoulder mobility is due to contractures of the muscles of the axilla and chest (see Ch. 2.)

Difficulty in abduction and flexion of the shoulder is best treated in my experience by surgical contracture releases and muscle transfers, which are soft tissue procedures. When there is loss of *passive* overhead movement that is significant, at around 150 degrees, surgery is indicated.

Treatment requires the **Modified Quad** surgery (see Ch. 2).

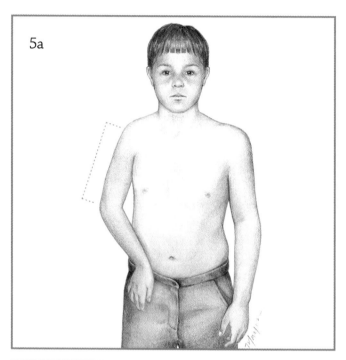

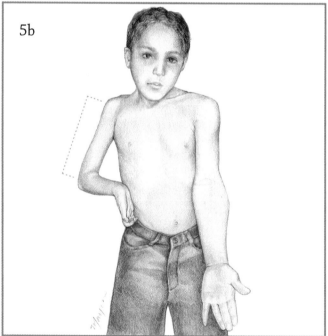

Question 5: Is the arm shorter? Diagnosis is made by directly measuring the upper arm from shoulder to elbow and comparing with the uninjured side (Figure 5.5a and 5.5b). A difference of greater than 20% may require surgery to lengthen. Lines mark areas of interest.

Treatment: Question 5

Severe shortening of the arm is functionally limiting, since full extension to match the other arm is not possible. This is primarily a bony problem and will require bone lengthening surgery to correct. The appropriate method is Ilizarov bone lengthening; in this surgery, an osteotomy cut is made in the humerus and allowed to partially heal. Metal rods placed on each side of the surgical cut are then gradually pulled apart, thereby stretching the bone and the limb. New bone will grow into the defect, resulting in lengthening of the extremity.

Several inches of length are achievable using the Ilizarov technique. If there is a rotation problem as well, that can be straightened with the Ilizarov procedure as long as no SHEAR is present.

Treatment requires the **Ilizarov** surgery (see Ch. 3).

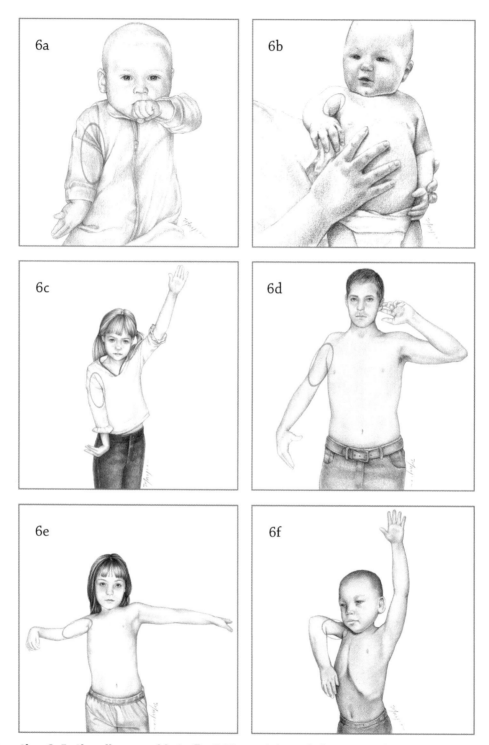

Question 6: Is the elbow unable to flex? Diagnosis is made by viewing the child's spontaneous (Figure 5.6a) or active (Figure 5.6b, 5.6c, 5.6d, 5.6e, 5.6f) attempts to flex the elbow. Note that in Figure 5.6e and 5.6f the child is using shoulder abduction to reduce the effects of gravity in an attempt to flex the elbow. The most common cause of elbow flexion weakness is actually co-contraction with the triceps, such that the triceps overpowers the biceps. BTX-A injection to the triceps is therefore the best way to treat this condition at any age. Nerve grafting should be reserved for the very severe cases (about 10% of those with clinical loss of elbow flexion). Circles mark areas of interest.

Treatment: Question 6

Loss of flexion of the elbow is a common problem in children with injury to the C6 nerve root. Most of the time this is due to co-contraction between the biceps and the triceps since the triceps is less affected by the injury, if at all. In infants, the treatment should be aimed at testing for the presence of co-contraction, and if this is present, then administration of BTX-A to the triceps has a favorable outcome. If there is such severe injury that the C6 root is completely injured, then nerve repair with grafting or nerve transfer may be required.

Treatment requires **BTX-A** injections or **Nerve Repair** surgery (see Chs. 1 and 2).

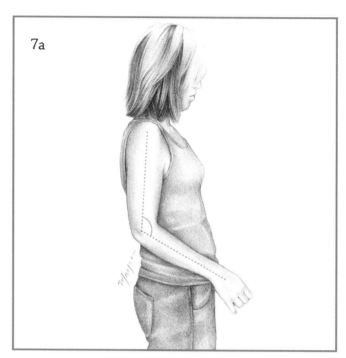

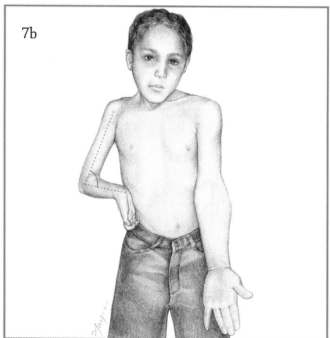

Question 7: Is there an elbow flexion contracture? Diagnosis is made by viewing the child's resting elbow position (Figure 5.7a, 5.7b). A fixed flexion contracture is obvious visually and a biceps tendon cord is palpable over the elbow crease; comparison with the uninjured side will show that no cord is palpable over that crease. Contractures over 15 degrees are significant and may require biceps tendon lengthening surgery. Splinting and serial casting do not typically have long-term efficacy. The most common cause of elbow flexion contracture is weakness in the triceps, such that the biceps overpowers the triceps. Lines mark areas of interest.

Treatment: Question 7

The presence of a fixed elbow contracture is usually caused by an overly strong biceps which is not balanced by an intact triceps. The root cause is a C7 injury which recovers less than the C6 root, or not at all.

There is some literature that discusses the use of BTX-A and casting in treatment of fixed elbow contractures, but in my experience, the best treatment is surgical lengthening of an overly tight biceps tendon (see Ch. 2.).

Treatment requires the use of **Biceps Tendon Lengthening** surgery (see Ch. 3).

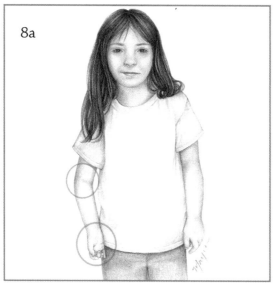

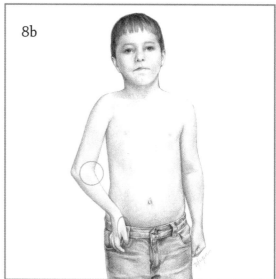

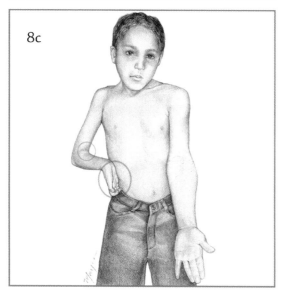

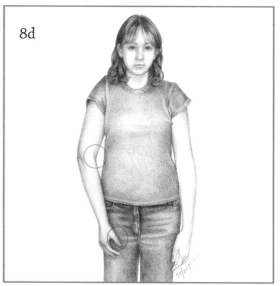

Question 8: Is the forearm supinated? This is an important determination that is made by carefully viewing the child's extremity position at rest. The upper arm may be in neutral (Figure 5.8a), in which case the elbow crease is fully visible (upper circle) and the forearm will appear to be supinated. Alternatively, and more commonly, medial rotation of the upper arm is present (upper circles in Figure 5.8b, 5.8c, 5.8d). Attention to the hand position compared with the uninjured side will show that the dorsum of the hand is not as visible on the injured side as on the uninjured side at rest (lower circles). In 5.8d, there is a supination deformity of the forearm present in the face of a medial rotation deformity of the arm (ARMS deformity, p. 39). This unusual variant is recognized by the fact that the first web space of the affected hand is visible at rest (lower circle). See also box in Chapter 3. Circles mark areas of interest.

Treatment: Question 8

Most patients with a brachial plexus injury sustained at birth will have a neutral or pronated posture of the forearm. However, it is possible to have the opposite situation, an overly supinated forearm.

After treating any medial rotation deformity of the shoulder, the supinated forearm is generally best treated with a forearm osteotomy. In this operation, the radius (and sometimes the ulna as well) are cut surgically and rotated into the neutral position.

Treatment requires the use of **Forearm Osteotomy** surgery (see Ch. 3).

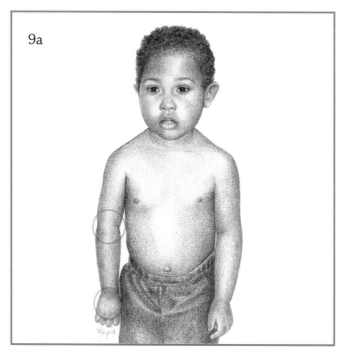

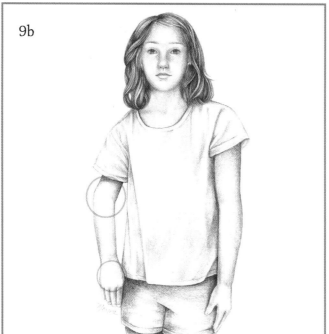

Question 9: Is the forearm pronated? This is an important determination that is made by carefully viewing the child's extremity position at rest. The upper arm is typically in medial rotation (upper circles show loss of elbow crease). Attention to the hand position compared with the uninjured side will show that the dorsum of the hand is more visible on the injured side compared to the uninjured side at rest (lower circles).

Treatment: Question 9

Most patients with a partially healed brachial plexus injury sustained at birth will have a neutral or pronated posture of the forearm. It is actually difficult to have a fixed pronation deformity although this does occur rarely. In general, the forearm is in neutral but is attached to a medially rotated arm, thus giving the appearance of a pronation posture.

After treating the medial rotation deformity of the shoulder, the forearm is generally "released" into a neutral position. Any residual pronation deformity can be treated with forearm osteotomy if significant (see Ch. 3).

Treatment requires the use of **Triangle Tilt** and/or **Forearm Osteotomy** surgery (see Ch. 3).

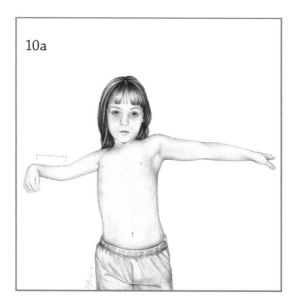

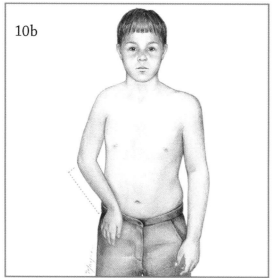

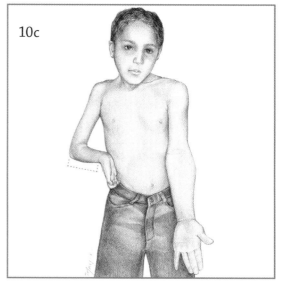

Question 10: Is the forearm shorter? In severe injuries, the arm and forearm length are decreased due to the nerve injury. Direct observation and measurement of the forearm compared with the uninjured side make the diagnosis. A difference of 30% is significant and may require surgical bony lengthening. Lines mark areas of interest.

Treatment: Question 10

Severe shortening of the forearm is functionally limiting, since full extension to match the other arm is not possible. This is primarily a bony problem and will require bone lengthening surgery to correct. The appropriate method is Ilizarov bone lengthening; in this surgery, an osteotomy cut is made in the radius and ulna bones of the forearm and allowed to partially heal. Metal rods placed on each side of the surgical cut are then gradually pulled apart, thereby stretching the bone and the limb. New bone will grow into the defect, resulting in lengthening of the extremity.

Several inches of length are achievable using the Ilizarov technique. If there is a rotation problem as well, that can also be straightened with an Ilizarov apparatus.

Treatment requires the **Ilizarov** surgery (see Ch. 3).

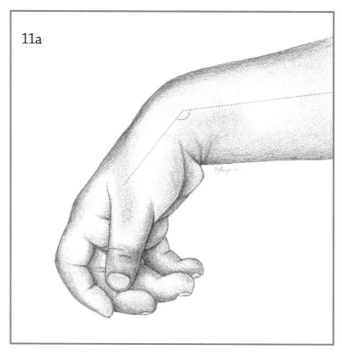

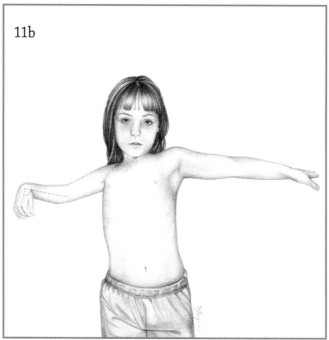

Question 11: Is the wrist dropped? In C7 injuries, the triceps and wrist and finger extensors are affected and a wrist drop is often seen. Direct observation and measurements of the wrist-forearm angle will make the diagnosis. Wrist injury can recover for up to several years. The patient must be monitored for the presence of flexion contractures which must be treated in longstanding wrist drop.

Treatment: Question 11

A wrist drop and loss of finger and thumb extension are due to a severe C7 nerve root injury. This may recover with time, up to 5 or 6 years, but if not, surgery is indicated. Tendon transfers, using healthy tendons from the flexor (volar) side of the forearm and hand, can restore at least some active wrist extension as well as finger extension and thumb opposition. These generally do not work well until the age of 6 to 7 years due to weakness in the tendon structure before that age. If earlier fixation is required, a tendon tightening (tenodesis) or wrist capsule tightening (capsulodesis) may be performed as a temporizing measure.

In some long-standing cases, a free muscle transfer surgery may add healthy muscle to help extend the wrist.

Treatment requires **Tendon Transfer** and sometimes **Free Gracilis Muscle Transfer** surgery.

15 QUESTIONS for OBPI Patient Evaluation

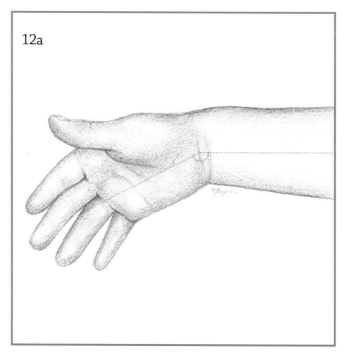

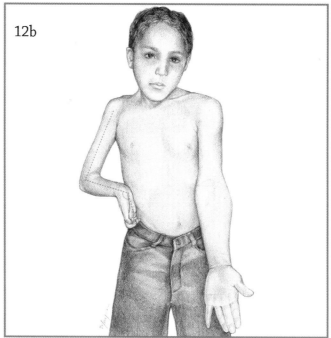

Question 12: Is the wrist ulnar-deviated? In some injuries, the wrist will deviate to the ulnar side, reflecting underlying muscle imbalances. Direct observation and measurements of the wrist-forearm angle will make the diagnosis. Wrist injury can recover for up to several years. Lines mark areas of interest.

Treatment: Question 12

Deviation of the wrist to the ulnar side of the forearm is common due to imbalances in the muscles and tendons supplying that area. This is generally treated by therapy and splinting, but in some cases, bony surgery to correct the length discrepancies between the radius (too long) and the ulna (too short) may be required.

Treatment requires **Forearm Wedge Osteotomy** surgery of the radius.

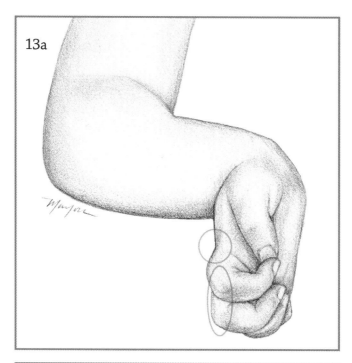

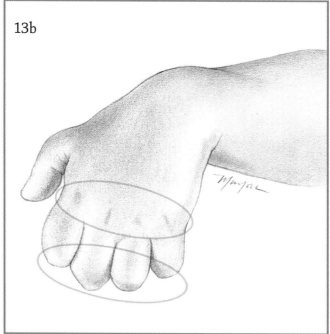

Question 13: Are the metacarpophalangeal (MCP) joints contracted? In severe injuries, the MCP joints will become stiff in extension (Figure 5.13a, 5.13b). Note that usually the proximal interphalangeal (PIP) joints are in flexion, reflecting underlying muscle imbalances. Direct observation of the fingers will make the diagnosis, along with palpation of excessive stiffness of the MCP joints. This is a difficult problem to treat and usually requires surgical release of the contractures. Circles mark areas of interest.

Treatment: Question 13

Tightness of the metacarpophalangeal (MCP) joints of the hand is due to a severe injury to the lower roots of the brachial plexus. Again, muscle imbalances cause the inability to flex the MCP joints. Initial treatment is aimed at loosening the MCP joints with a combination of passive stretches and night time dynamic splinting.

Ultimately, surgery to release the tight ligaments of the MCP joints may be required, followed by intensive therapy and splinting. There is a high rate of recurrence of this deformity, emphasizing the severe consequences of injury to the lower roots of the brachial plexus (see Ch. 1).

Treatment requires **Metacarpophalangeal Joint Collateral Ligament Release** surgery followed by intensive therapy and splinting.

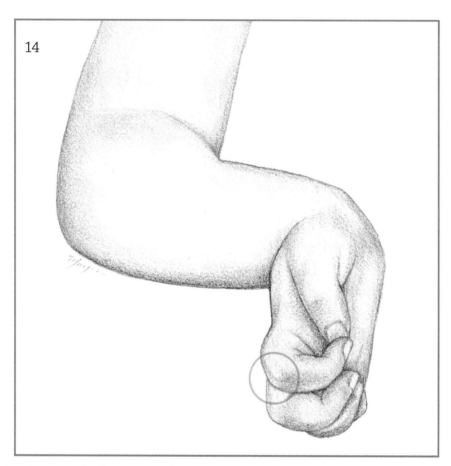

14

Question 14: Are the fingers paralyzed? In severe injuries, the fingers will not flex (Figure 5.14). Note that usually the metacarpophalangeal (MCP) joints are in extension and stiff, while the proximal interphalangeal (PIP) joints are in flexion and supple. Complete finger paralysis will require reanimation of the fingers through advanced surgical techniques. Direct observation of the fingers will make the diagnosis, along with palpation of excessive stiffness of the MCP joints and lack of active flexion of the fingers. Circle marks area of interest.

Treatment: Question 14

Loss of finger flexion is a devastating consequence of brachial plexus injury in children. There is a lack of nerve supply to the forearm and hand as well as terminal atrophy of the muscles of the forearm and hand. There is no therapy that can address this situation. Major surgery to restore both nerve supply and muscle is required.

The first stage of supplying nerve is done by transferring part of the nerve supply of the opposite brachial plexus (contralateral C7 nerve transfer). The second stage transfers a gracilis muscle from the inner thigh to replace the lost muscle of the forearm, and to perform the function of closing the fingers and wrist. This is a very complex surgery, requiring the services of 3 to 4 specialists within the operating room. This emphasizes the severe consequences of injury to the lower roots of the brachial plexus (see Ch. 1).

Treatment requires **Contralateral C7 Nerve Transfer and Free Functional Gracilis Muscle Transfer** surgery followed by intensive therapy and splinting.

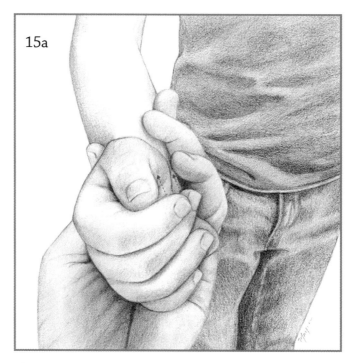

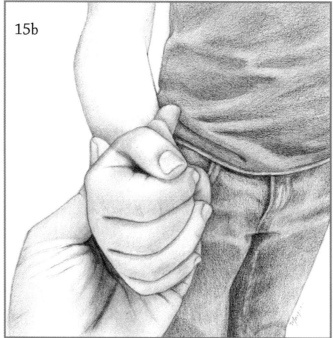

Question 15: Do the fingers move, but poorly? In severe injuries, the fingers will flex weakly (Figure 5.15a, 5.15b). Many if not most cases of finger weakness are due to MCP contractures, and should be treated as such (Figure 5.13). Direct observation of the fingers will make the diagnosis, along with palpation of excessive stiffness of the MCP joints and weakness in active flexion of the fingers. Arrows mark areas of interest.

Treatment: Question 15

Weakness of finger flexion is a devastating consequence of brachial plexus injury in children. There is a lack of nerve supply to the forearm and hand as well as significant atrophy of the muscles of the forearm and hand. The main cause of finger flexion loss in cases where some finger movement is visible, is tightness of the metacarpophalangeal (MCP) joints of the hand. Treatment is aimed at loosening the MCP joints with a combination of passive stretches and night time dynamic splinting.

Ultimately, surgery to release the tight ligaments of the MCP joints may be required, followed by intensive therapy and splinting. There is a high rate of recurrence of this deformity, emphasizing the severe consequences of injury to the lower roots of the brachial plexus (see Ch. 1).

Treatment requires **Metacarpophalangeal Joint Collateral Ligament Release** surgery followed by intensive therapy and splinting.

Application of the 15 questions system

Prior to evaluation by the "15 questions" system, patients are classified by two parameters, age and previous surgeries. The age classifications are: 0-3 months, 3-6 months, 6-12 months, 12-18 months, 18-24 months, 2 years – 6 years, 12 years – 20 years and 20 years +. Previous nerve-, muscle-and bone-related surgeries are documented.

The fifteen questions are used to describe the position and growth of rigid elements and joint movements in the upper extremity. By describing alterations in function, all of the elements that are affected by the injury, including nerve, muscle and bone are encompassed by this system.

The questions are listed from above downward anatomically which is the most efficient way to evaluate the extremity clinically. The system is organized in this chapter by describing the appropriate physical examination on the left sided pages and the treatment outline on the facing right sided pages. In this way, I hope that an organized, logical evaluation and treatment plan may be constructed for each individual patient. I believe that this will account for the unique nature of each individual injury but still take advantage of knowledge of common patterns that exist beneath each clinical presentation.

On my current website, there is also a section that allows caregivers to send in completed "15 Questions" forms that I can comment on in terms of a treatment plan for the patient entered: http://drnathbrachialplexus.com/referral.

Finally, Table 5.I lists the most common patterns of clinical presentation for patients using the "15 Questions" format. This can be compared to the individual child's data and will allow immediate feedback on a suggested treatment plan.

Table 5.I. *Common Patterns Using the "15 Questions" Format*

Pattern	Treatment
1 only	Scapular shaving (ostectomy), if severe
1+2	Triangle Tilt surgery + ostectomy
1+2+3+4	Mod Quad surgery + Triangle Tilt surgery+ ostectomy
1+2+6	Botulinum toxin/nerve repair + Triangle Tilt surgery+ostectomy
1+2+3+4+6	Botulinum toxin/nerve repair + Mod Quad surgery + Triangle Tilt surgery + ostectomy
3+4	Mod Quad surgery
3+4+6	Botulinum toxin/nerve repair + Mod Quad surgery
1+2+7	Triangle Tilt surgery + ostectomy + biceps tendon lengthening
1+2+3+4+7	Mod Quad surgery + Triangle Tilt surgery + ostectomy + biceps tendon lengthening
11	Wrist and finger tendon transfers

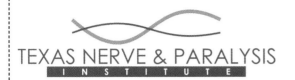

Texas Nerve & Paralysis Institute
2201 W. Holcombe Blvd. Ste. 225
Houston, Texas 77030
Scheduling: (713) 592-9900
Fax: (713) 592-9921

Patient Name _____ DOB _____ SSN _____

Patient Phone # _____ Insurance _____

Referring Physician _____ Phone _____ Fax _____

Diagnosis _____

Appointment Date and Time _____

http://www.drnathmedical.com/referral

Age

- ☐ 0 - 3 months
- ☐ 3 - 6 months
- ☐ 6 - 12 months
- ☐ 12 - 18 months
- ☐ 18 - 24 months
- ☐ 2 years to 12 years
- ☐ 12+ years

Previous Surgery

- ☐ Primary (Nerve Grafting) _____
- ☐ Mod Quad _____
- ☐ Triangel Tilt _____
- ☐ Humeral Osteotomy _____
- ☐ Wrist/Hand Tendon Transfers _____

* Please indicate surgeon in the space provided. *

Comments

_____

_____

_____

_____

_____

_____

_____

_____

Signature _____ Date

15 QUESTIONS

1. Is the SCAPULA Elevated? ☐

2. Is the ARM Internally Rotated? ☐

3. Is the SHOULDER AROM <120 Degrees? ☐

4. Is the SHOULDER PROM <150 Degrees? ☐

5. Is the ARM Shorter? ☐

6. Is the ELBOW Unable to Flex? ☐

7. Is there an ELBOW Flexion Contracture? ☐

8. Is the FOREARM Supinated? ☐

9. Is the FOREARM Pronated? ☐

10. Is the FOREARM Shorter? ☐

11. Is the WRIST Dropped? ☐

12. Is the WRIST Ulnar deviated? ☐

13. Are the MCP Joints Contracted? ☐

14. Are the Fingers Paralyzed? ☐

15. Do the FINGERS Move, but Poorly? ☐

Notes

Notes

Glenoid fossa (continued)
    retroversion, 28
Glenoid version, 41, **53**, 54
Gracilis muscle. See Surgery.
Growth, **6**, 7, 39, 41

H

Horner's sign, 9
Humeral derotational osteotomy. See
    surgery.
Humeral head, **36**, **37**, **42**
    anterior dislocation, 41
    impingement upon, **39**, **40**, 41, **42**, 53
    inferior dislocation. 25, 28
    medial rotation, 9, 39
    posterior dislocation, 37, 39
    subluxation. See Subluxation,
        humeral.
Humeral subluxation. See Subluxation,
    humeral.
Humerus, 5, **36**, 38

I

Ilizarov. See surgery.
Infraspinatus muscle, 7, **20**, 21, **26**
Internal rotator muscles (internal rotators).
    See Shoulder.

K

Klumpke's paralysis, 7

L

Latissimus dorsi muscle, 9, 25, **26**, **27**, 28,
    29, 30, 37
Long thoracic nerve, 2, **5**, 9
Luxury innervation, 12

M

Magnetic resonance imaging (MRI), 11, 40,
    41
    positional, **40**, 43
    upright, **40**
Mallet. See Modified Mallet System and
    Nath modification.
MCP (metacarpophalangeal) joint. See
    Deformity.
Medial rotation. See Shoulder.
Medial rotation contracture (MRC). See
    Deformity.
Median nerve, **14**, 20
Mesoneurium, 2

Metacarpophalangeal (MCP) joint. See
    Deformity.
Microneurolysis (neurolysis). See Surgery.
Mod Quad surgery. See Surgery.
Modified Mallet system, 22, 40, 46, 54
    Nath modification, 22, **23**
Modified Quad surgery. See Surgery
Motor learning therapy. See Therapy.
MRC (medial rotation contracture). See
    Deformity.
MRI. See Magnetic resonance imaging.
Muscle, 20
    co-contraction(s), 7, 8, 10, 21, 22, 25,
        41, 70, 71
    contracture(s), 8, 10, 11, 21, 22, 26, 27,
        28, 36, 61, 65, 67, 72, 73, 80, 84
    denervated, 7, 8, 12, 21
    imbalance(s), 7, 8, 21, 22
    opposing, 7, 21, **25**
    transfers. See Surgery.
Musculocutaneous nerve, **14**, 26

N

Narakas. See Classification of injury.
NCV (nerve conduction velocity). See
    Nerve.
Nerve, 2, 3
    conduction, 2, 3, 11, 12, 13, 28
    conduction velocity (NCV), 11
    decompression. See Surgery.
    healing, 3, 4, 6, 9, 12, 13, 21
    in-continuity, **3**, **4**, 9, 12
    fascicle, 2, 3, 4
    fibers, 2
    grafting. See Surgery.
    motor, 2, 3, 11
    peripheral, 2
    reconstruction. See Surgery.
    recovery, 3, 4, **6**, 7, 9, 10, 22
    regeneration, 3, 4, 9, 11, 12
    rupture, **4**, 7, 9, 11, 13
    transfer. See Surgery.
Nervous system, 2, 9
Neurapraxia, **3**, 5, 9
Neuroanatomy, 2
Neurolysis. See Surgery.
Neuroma, 4, **13**
Neuromuscular anatomy, 20
Neuron, 2, 9
Neurotization. See Surgery.
Neurotmesis, **3**, 4, 9
Neurotoxin. See Botulinum Toxin A.

O

OBPI. See Obstetric brachial plexus injury.
Obstetric brachial plexus injuries (OBPI),
    4, 6, 10
    associated injuries, 5
    location and severity of, 5, **6**, 7, 8, 9,
        11
    rate, 4
    risk factor, 4
Ostectomy. See Surgery.
Osteotomy. See Surgery.

P

Paralysis(es), 7, 9, 22, 28, 86
Paraspinal muscle, 7, 11
Pectoralis muscle, 25, **26**, **27**, 28, 29, 30, 37,
    41
Perineurium, 2
Phrenic nerve, 9, 12
PIP (proximal interphalangeal) joint. See
    Deformity.
Posterior glenohumeral capsulorrhaphy.
    See Surgery.
Prognosis, 4, 10
PROM (passive range of motion) exercises
    See Range of motion exercises.
Proximal interphalangeal (PIP) joint. See
    Deformity.
Pseudoglenoid. See Glenoid fossa.

Q

Quad surgery. See Surgery.

R

Radial nerve, **5**, 20
Radius, 75, 79, 83
Range of motion (ROM) exercises, 14, 23,
    24, 41
Rhomboid muscles, 7, 8, 9, **20**, 61
ROM exercises. See Range of motion
    exercises.
Rotator cuff, 9, 21, 26, 27, 28
Rotator muscles
    internal. See Shoulder.
    external. See Shoulder.

S

Scapula
    acromion. See Acromion.
    anatomy, **36**